Psychiatric Nursing

Person to Person

USING NURSING MODELS SERIES

General Editors:

Jane E Schober SRN, RCNT, DipN Ed, DipN (Lond), RNT
Lecturer, Nursing Studies, Institute of Advanced Nursing Education,
Royal College of Nursing

Christine Webb BA, MSc, PhD, SRN, RSCN, RNT
Principal Lecturer in Nursing, Department of Nursing, Health and
Applied Social Studies, Bristol Polytechnic, Bristol

The views expressed in this book are those of the authors of individual chapters
and do not necessarily reflect the opinions of the series editors.

Psychiatric Nursing

Person to Person

Blair Collister
MSc, RMN, RGN, DN, DANS, RCNT, RNT

Lecturer in Nursing
University of Manchester
Department of Nursing

Edward Arnold

A division of Hodder & Stoughton

LONDON   BALTIMORE   MELBOURNE   AUCKLAND

© 1988 Blair Collister

First published in Great Britain 1988

British Library Cataloguing in Publication Data

Psychiatric Nursing.
    I. Psychiatric patient. Nursing
    I. Collister, Blair
    II. Series
    610.73′68

    ISBN 0 340 41772 2

Typeset by Wearside Tradespools, Fulwell, Sunderland
Printed and bound in Great Britain for Edward Arnold, the educational,
academic and medical publishing division of Hodder & Stoughton
Limited, 41 Bedford Square, London WC1 3DQ by
Anchor Brendan Ltd, Tiptree, Essex

Contents

List of Contributors

Blair Collister MSc, RMN, SRN, RNT is a lecturer in the Department of Nursing, University of Manchester. He completed his nurse training in the Isle of Man and subsequently worked as a tutor at Rainhill Hospital, Liverpool, before taking up his present post in 1982.

Bill Lemmer RMN, DipN, Dip Psycho-Social and Family-Centred Nursing (Cassel Hospital), Dip Ed (London), RNT is a Staff Development Tutor at the Nightingale School, London. He has conducted a 3 year research project into the management of change in mental health care and is reading for a Master of Philosophy degree at the University of Surrey.

Meg Miller SRN, RMN, DipN Ed, DipN is a tutor at St Mary's Hospital, Paddington, London. She teaches aspects of mental health to RGN learners throughout their training as well as during the mental health module.

Ian Moore RMN is a Staff Nurse on the Acute Unit at St Clement's Hospital, Ipswich.

Sue Ritter MA, SRN, RMN, is Senior Nurse (Research) at the Bethlem Royal and Maudsley Hospitals. She read English and American Literature at university before doing her General Nurse training at St Thomas' Hospital. She began her RMN training in 1977, and worked as a Charge Nurse for six years at the Maudsley Hospital before taking up her present job in 1986.

Gary Rix BSc, RMN is a Nurse Researcher in the Dennis Hill Regional Secure Unit, Bethlem Royal Hospital, Kent.

Felicity Stockwell SRN, RMN, RNT is a Tutor at Whittingham Hospital, near Preston, Lancashire. She is the author of *The Unpopular Patient* and *The Nursing Process in Psychiatric Nursing*.

Ben Thomas BSc (Hons), MSc, SRN, RMN, RNT was formerly a Staff Nurse with West Glamorgan Health Authority. He is now a tutor at the Maudsley Hospital.

Mike Thomas RMN is a Charge Nurse within the Elderly Services Team at Prestwich Hospital, Manchester. He previously worked as a Staff Nurse at Leigh Infirmary, Manchester and at Leighton Hospital, Crewe.

Verina Wilde BNurs, SRN, HV Cert, NDN Cert, RMN, RNT is a tutor at Macclesfield School of Nursing. She previously worked as a Behavioural Nurse Therapist in Macclesfield and as a Sister at the Mersey Regional Adolescent Psychiatric Unit, and recently completed the MSc (Nursing) course at the University of Manchester.

Preface

This book represents another step in the process of evaluation of nursing models. It does so by reporting the efforts of psychiatric nurses who have attempted to integrate models into their everyday nursing practice in a conscious and deliberative way. Contributors have each selected an approach relevant to their own practice, and have given an account of their experience in the form of a care plan and discussion.

It should be pointed out that some of the models employed may not be regarded as *nursing* models *per se*, because they would not be found in the usual literature on nursing models. However, their inclusion can be justified on at least two counts. In the first place these chapters all represent 'models used by nurses' and, since nursing models are precisely that, then all these models have relevance for nurses. In the second place, the chapters represent a considered, deliberate decision about the kind of nursing practice in which contributors see themselves participating, and the way in which that practice can be framed. Thus, although in some chapters you may not find references to well-known nurse theorists, what you may well find is an approach to patient care which approximates to your own view of what nursing practice is all about.

I first became aware of the existence of nursing models in the late 1970s as a postgraduate nursing student at the University of Manchester. My recollection of that time is that I was discovering a lot of new ideas (not only related to nursing models), almost all of which I found to be intuitively right. In effect I was a sort of 'ideas dustbin', and I accepted uncritically nearly everything I read.

However, the opportunity to discuss, challenge and debate the issues with teaching staff and with my fellow students encouraged me to recognise two things. Firstly, I had opinions and ideas of my own, which have been developing and changing ever since. Secondly, the ideas I had read were (and are) written by human beings like you and me, and we are perfectly entitled to accept or reject these ideas as we think fit. But the decision to accept or reject a particular view must be an *informed* decision,

based on a thorough understanding of the ideas and not on ignorance or prejudice.

My own understanding of nursing models has continued to develop through teaching undergraduate and postgraduate students, presenting papers and attending conferences, and through my appointment as an External Assessor for Unit 3 of the London University Diploma in Nursing. This understanding is, I feel, growing all the time. My own ideas about nursing practice are also changing constantly through contact with patients in a variety of clinical settings as part of my day-to-day work. Finally, my (imperfect) understanding has been influenced by the work involved in editing this book.

It would have been possible to discuss the application of models in psychiatric nursing in a series of chapters each focusing on a diagnostic category such as paranoid schizophrenia or mania. However, it was felt that this would betray a primary goal, that of examining patient-centred nursing care within the framework of nursing models. Instead, each chapter looks at a particular patient problem because we believe that certain problems may be experienced by patients irrespective of their medical diagnosis. Although the term used to denote some problems may be that of a medical diagnosis (for example depression or anxiety) it is emphasised that these terms refer to the constellation of thoughts, feelings and behaviour manifested by the patient. This is in contrast to the aetiology, signs and symptoms, treatment and prognosis which would be the focus if the terms were used medically.

In several instances, the nursing assessment reveals problems in addition to the one which is the focus of the chapter. Discussion will to some extent ignore these problems unless they are of a high priority, but the care plans will indicate the appropriate goals and nursing action for these subsidiary problems.

Each contributor is an experienced psychiatric nurse and each chapter reveals the quality of interpersonal skills which are brought to the nurse–patient relationship. Also, since each is sharing his or her experience, it is hoped that the reader will experience a sense of dialogue with the writer. These two aspects capture the interpersonal nature of this work, and together form the reason for the subtitle on the cover of this book: *Person to Person*.

Blair Collister
Manchester, 1987

Note: Throughout this book the pronoun *she* refers to the nurse or carer and *he* to the patient or client. This distinction is made for the sake of clarity only and no bias is intended.

Acknowledgements

I wish to thank the many people who have contributed, both directly and indirectly, to the work in this book. Most of them would not be aware of their influence, and it would not be possible to name them all. They include:

Those with whom I have shared my working life
  The staff and patients of Ballamona and Noble's Hospitals, Isle of Man
  Erstwhile colleagues at Rainhill Hospital, Prescot
  Present and former colleagues in the University of Manchester Department of Nursing
  Students of nursing whom it has been, and continues to be, my privilege to teach
Those who have so readily shared in the writing of this book
  The contributors
  Christine Webb, Series Editor
Those who share my life
  Mary, Damion and Sinead

In Memory of:
  My Mother, who died about the time this book was finished, and the late Joyce Fernandes, who typed my contribution.

I

Introduction: sharing perceptions

Blair Collister

The range of nursing models facing nurses today is bewildering both in terms of numbers and in the scope of their usefulness. In preparing to write this introductory chapter it crossed my mind to consult a variety of texts and to count the number of models reported. Then I could have started this paragraph with a punchy statement detailing the precise number of models which I had encountered. Caution prevailed. If I had done so, what reaction would I have been looking for? The commonest two would probably have been 'so what?', or a suitable expletive followed by the closing of this book! So I decided not to produce an impressive statistic, not least because I could not justify such a pointless exercise. Also, my understanding of the general idea of models (not just in nursing) leads me to believe that models help us to make sense of reality. Each of us has a model of nursing – a mental image – so the spurious statistic I was seeking is that there are as many models of nursing as there are nurses.

With so many models, some decision needs to be made about which of them may be useful, and some sort of consensus is required to unify our approach to practice and to avoid the emergence of a conceptual Tower of Babel.

In order for this to happen, it is necessary for nurses to develop an awareness of their own view of nursing. This involves, amongst other things, examining and discussing models developed by others so that the general idea of models can be understood and these models can be tested to see what, if anything, they have to offer our own practice. This book is intended to encourage that process.

This chapter introduces some background ideas by examining one aspect of nursing models and discussing the kinds of model which have influenced psychiatric nursing practice.

Metaphors in models

In this book, as in others in the series, each chapter contains an outline of the model which the writer has selected. Included in each outline is an indication of what the particular model has to say about *the person*. Here, three examples are given by way of illustration.

For Orem (1980) the healthy individual is a self-care agent, capable of responding to therapeutic self-care demands. These demands can be categorised according to the self-care requisites which they serve. Another view is offered by Roy (1980) for whom the person is an adaptive system. Through the cognator and regulator mechanisms stimuli are interpreted and the adaptive response occurs through four adaptive modes. Finally, Johnson (1980) conceptualises the individual as a behavioural system. The behaviour of the person is classified according to behavioural subsystems and the goals of this behaviour are equilibrium and system survival.

Although it is not the main point of this discussion, it may be worth commenting on the jargon or vocabulary used by nurse theorists, and the labels they use for various concepts. It seems that the jargon used by nurse theorists is no better nor worse than the terms encountered – and used – by nurses elsewhere. (Don't believe it? What about gustatory hallucinations, the festinant gait or the primary delusion?) Experience suggests that if nurses meet an unfamiliar medical term in a patient's case notes, they will be prompted to look up the meaning of the word. Responsibility is accepted for the knowledge gap and the nurse responds appropriately. Paradoxically, if a nurse meets an unfamiliar term when reading about a nursing model then the tendency seems to be to project the inadequacy onto the writer. Whilst this may be justifiable in cases where the writer has not offered an adequate description or definition, the significance of these two different reactions lies in their indication of what nurses perceive to be important. Medical knowledge and medical terms are seen to be more important and relevant to nursing practice. This raises two issues, which relate to the relevance of the medical model to nursing practice and the idea of authority based on expert knowledge. These issues will be discussed later in this chapter.

To return to the three descriptions of the person. What is at issue is not the jargon used, but how these ideas are interpreted and incorporated into practice. Theory which is applied to a practice discipline may come from one of two sources. On the one hand, the theory may be developed, through research, from nursing practice itself. On the other hand, theory from another discipline may be taken and applied to nursing.

In either case, the intention is usually to describe and explain nursing in a way that makes sense to the writer and to the reader. In effect, the theorist is saying 'If we think of the person *as* a —, then this may help us to understand the human processes at work. It may also help us to make decisions about nursing care.' In order for readers to understand the description and discussion which would follow this opening statement, it is important that they remember that this is an exercise in imagination.

However, what tends to happen is that the ideas are used in a very concrete fashion, often to the detriment of understanding because the theoretical

framework itself is not fully developed and cannot completely explain the situation which it represents. As a consequence, when a particular model is used, it is assumed that the person actually *is* a behavioural system, or a self-care agent or an adaptive system. Two consequences of this emerge. The first is that, because of the incomplete development of the model, nurses are unable to analyse and understand the situation and hence are unable to assess, plan, implement and evaluate care within the framework of the model. The second and more significant consequence is that the metaphor of nursing models is not appreciated. That is, a particular model may be presented in a way which says, 'the person is an adaptive system', instead of saying 'in certain circumstance, the person may be viewed *as if* she or he were an adaptive system'. The circumstances referred to are the assumptions and values underlying the model, and the important thing is that they may not always apply. Also, the 'as if' is ignored. The person is not viewed as if they were 'like', or 'similar to' whatever the concept is, but they are taken to *be* that concept. A similar argument could be developed for the concepts 'nursing', 'health' and 'environment' as described by a particular model.

The medical model

This idea of a metaphor being used to explain reality is not new to psychiatric nurses. Several writers including Szasz (1960) have pointed to the inappropriate application of the term 'sick' as a metaphor for psychological disturbance. The argument goes something like this: systematic observation of emotionally and behaviourally disturbed individuals revealed similarities between individuals (Kraepelin, 1906; Bleuler, 1911). It has been suggested that sense could be made of these similarities if the people were thought of as being 'ill'. If the person were thought of as suffering from illness then it would be possible to elicit aetiological factors and signs and symptoms indicating a particular illness which could be diagnosed. Subsequent work concentrated on identifying and describing these factors and developing a diagnostic classification. However, this went on at a time when the consequences of such a process were not apparent or available. The diagnosis of physical illness led to predictive statements about prognosis, the prescription of appropriate treatments, and to cure, but this was not the case with mental illness. Few treatments were available and cure could not be anticipated except by allowing some diseases, in some individuals, to run their course. In this context it is worth noting that the prognostic implications for a group of people diagnosed today as schizophrenic are little different from those of a similar group of people who would have been diagnosed 70 years ago as suffering from dementia praecox.

Generally, of each group about a half would get better either marginally or completely and the other half would remain the same or get worse (Bleuler, 1911; Brown *et al.*, 1972; Hoenig and Hamilton, 1966; Simon *et al.*, 1965). Thus, despite the range of diagnostic tools and medical treatments developed during the past half century, the same

proportion of schizophrenics will recover as 70 years ago.

Another problem with the concept 'diagnosis' in psychiatry is the inconsistency of the outcome of the diagnostic process employed by psychiatrists. As a consequence of this inconsistency, the same signs and symptoms may lead to different diagnoses being made by different psychiatrists.

A further confusion arises when the assumption is made that mental illness is present even in the absence of the appropriate 'clinical picture'. In this situation, a 'type two' error (Scheff, 1967) is made. What happens is that a psychiatrist is confronted by an individual with some sort of problem. If there is no evidence *to the contrary*, then mental illness is presumed to be present. Various differential diagnoses are made, and the appropriate treatment is prescribed.

As a consequence of these inconsistencies and confusions in diagnosis and treatment in psychiatry, the process indicated in Fig. 1.1 will operate. Other

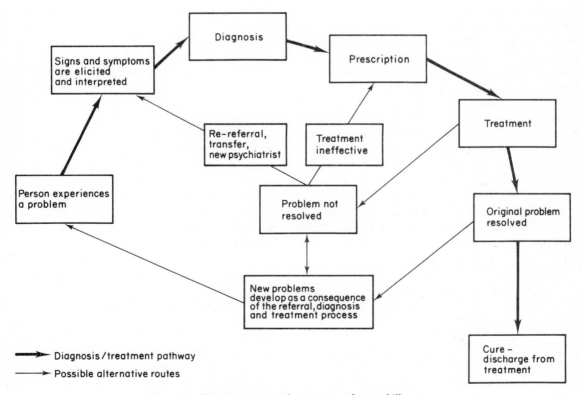

Fig. 1.1 The diagnosis and treatment of mental illness

views of mental illness have been discussed elsewhere (Collister, 1986) and an analysis of the consequences of the inappropriate application of the medical model is offered by Hargie and McCartan (1986).

Two points emerge from this outline of models of mental illness. The first is that psychiatric nurses are familiar with situations in which more than one view, or model, operates and may therefore be said to have an advantage over nurses in some other specialities. This is not least because psychiatric nurses will be aware of the drawbacks when a model is inadequate in its scope and does not encompass all the factors which operate, and of the implications for nursing action when one model is substituted for another.

The second point, germane to this introductory chapter, is that the case of mental illness illustrates how the over-elaborate and exclusive application of the metaphor to a particular situation often serves to confuse rather than clarify, and to divert attention away from other avenues of enquiry which may be of greater significance.

What is required of nurses, then, is that they should understand any model which they apply and in the process of application should be alert to the overall implications and the values underlying any model.

Notwithstanding uncertainties over diagnosis, there is another implication of ascribing the label 'illness' to the kind of problems experienced by the people with whom psychiatric nurses have contact.

Freidson (1970) states

> The medical profession has first claim to jurisdiction over the label of illness and anything to which it may be attached, irrespective of its ability to deal with it effectively. (p.251)

This raises the issue of power between professional groups and between professionals and their clients. The lip-service paid by psychiatrists to a 'multidisciplinary team' approach, and the reluctance of some to involve patients in decisions about care and treatment, is familiar to many nurses.

Sim (1981) says

> The 'team system' has eroded the psychiatrist's judgement and influence.... (p.437)

Sim's discussion is in defence of a positive approach to the management of the suicidal patient. However, the values underpinning his approach and the perceived relationship of psychiatry to other disciplines is further revealed by the following:

> The increasing responsibility of non-medical staff for patient care has handed over to other professionals very sick people who need continuous psychiatric diagnosis and treatment but who are retained tenaciously in entirely inappropriate programmes. (pp.437–438)

Since many nursing models, and the philosophy underpinning the nursing process, include the idea of patient's having a say in their care then the implications of the foregoing are self-evident.

The way in which interprofessional power is distributed is discussed by Strauss *et al.* (1964) and the strategies employed by attendants in opposition to medical decisions are identified by Scheff (1967).

What is at issue here, however, is the need for nurses to be aware of the political dimension of models in practice. This reflects Rogers' (1978) reference to 'political in a new sense'. Rogers describes his increasing awareness of the politics of interpersonal relationships. In this sense, *politics* refers to *power*, and of concern are the strategies which may be used to gain this power, who has the power to make decisions, and the consequences of these decisions. Even though nurses may wish to create a situation in which self-determination is vested with the patient, other interests could conspire to prevent this. The application of a particular model therefore goes beyond understanding a few unfamiliar words and changing the ward documentation.

A model of models

The dichotomy between the abstract representation of nursing offered by nurse theorists and the reality experienced by nurses may be explained, at least in part, by the metaphorical nature of models referred to earlier. Nurse theorists are attempting to develop an overall view of nursing – a metaparadigm. With further development and refining, it may then be possible to make statements which can be tested in reality to see if they hold true. In other words, it may be possible to formulate hypotheses which can be investigated through research. If, through rigorous testing, a statement is found to hold true in every situation in which it can reasonably be applied, then (and only then) it can be stated as a law. The type of theory which can be applied to *every* situation which it seeks to explain is termed nomothetic.

In nursing, some writers have taken theoretical perspectives from elsewhere and applied them to nursing. These include developmental theory, general systems theory, and stress-adaptation theory. Occasionally more than one of these perspectives is incorporated into a nursing model. In taking this approach it is assumed that the laws and relationships inherent in the adopted theory still hold good in its application in nursing.

Let us leave that for a moment and look at one interaction between a nurse (you) and a patient. In this interaction the nurse is likely to have a good idea about what to say and do; what to pay attention to and what to ignore; the possible response of the patient; and the likely outcome of the interaction. Thus the nurse has a theory, based on personal knowledge and experience, for this one interaction. This theory, which explains one (and only one) event, is termed idiothetic.

However, things may not go as expected and the theory may require modification for the nurse to feel confident about subsequent interactions with the same patient. Further modification of this 'theory of nursing' will take place through subsequent interactions with this patient and with other patients, with colleagues, and with changes in the nurse's knowledge and experience. However, we still have a theory which is limited in scope and only explains one nurse's view of the whole world of nursing. It could still be regarded as idiothetic since it only explains individual examples of the phenomenon 'nursing'. This idiothetic image represents what Fawcett (1984) refers to as a 'private image', and in many ways could be said to resemble the models used in this book.

In the process just described, rather than taking a theoretical perspective from outside nursing, the nurse has developed a theory based on observation and interpretation. Through repeated testing in reality it is modified and refined. Although we may not be aware of it, this is the process whereby we make sense of life in general, and not just nursing.

Thus, there are two processes of theory development, and these are described in detail by Dickoff and James (1968). The first, in which *existing* theory is used to explain the phenomenon under scrutiny, is termed inductive. The second, in which the phenomenon is observed, information collected and interpreted and a theory generated, is called deductive. In either case, the theory may require modification and interpretation to fit reality.

This adaptation and modification is a necessary part of theory development, and it is with this spirit of enquiry and challenge that nurses should approach the whole idea of models in nursing. It is suggested that each model referred to in this book is in a sense idiothetic since it represents one nurse's view of nursing.

The value of models lies in the idea that, as Ruddock (1972) suggests, they occupy the middle ground between an individual example (one nursing event) and a metaparadigm (a theory which explains the whole of nursing). Thus, although a writer may say that a particular model works with any patient in any setting, nurses may well find that interpretation, modification and elaboration is necessary to fit the model to reality. Hey presto, what was held to be nomothetic turns out to be idiothetic.

Ruddock puts this point elegantly, in quoting Kluckhohn and Murray (1949). He suggests that three standpoints are possible, represented by the following statements.

Every person is in certain respects

(a)   like all other people;
(b)   like some other people;
(c)   like no other person.

The view represented by statement (c) is idiothetic, since it refers the uniqueness of the individual. Statement (a) on the other hand is nomothetic, and it enables hypotheses to be made which can be applied to *all* people. However the point that

Ruddock is making is that the middle ground, represented by statement (b), is often overlooked, may be the most fruitful area for investigation and is the position occupied by models in the social sciences.

Two final points about the development and application of models are worth mentioning.

Several writers including Aggleton and Chalmers (1984) suggest that nursing models are the product of painstaking research and exploration. This is not always the case, at least in the earlier stages of their development. Discussion with writers including King, Roy and Orem reveals that each had known, in their thinking, research and practice, at least one episode of insight – an AHA! experience. This does not diminish the value of such an experience, but it is worth noting that some of the research and investigation came after (rather than before) the event.

The second point concerns the practical application of these ideas and has, I believe, implications for the way in which these ideas are presented to practitioners. King (1985) states unequivocally that theories are not applied in practice. *It is the knowledge derived from theory which is applied in practice.* Theories and models do not have a life of their own and if the knowledge is not explicated then they are valueless. Earlier, reference was made to the medical model. When I embarked on my training, no one said 'we use the biomedical model of mental illness', and this model was not represented as a discrete entity. No one said 'here is the biomedical model, learn it and use it in nursing practice'. What did happen, I now know with an Honours degree in Hindsight, was that I was taught the knowledge and skills necessary to practise as a nurse within the biomedical framework.

The observations I made on patients were to do with recognising and reporting signs and symptoms. With a few exceptions, my interactions were orientated to medical treatments rather than to a broader therapeutic approach. This is not to say that I did not form interpersonal relationships. I feel that I did, but what I question is the *goal* of the 'therapeutic use of self' which I believe I employed.

It is only with the hindsight just referred to that I am aware of what took place. There was no 'rote learning' of a model to be framed in practice. Rather, every aspect of practice and training was underpinned by this framework, and even questions on RMN State Finals papers were to do with listing signs and symptoms and describing the nurse's role in treatment.

Nurse educators (of which I am one) would do well to recognise this discrepancy between then and now. It is the knowledge and skills implicit in or derived from the model which constitute the content of nursing curricula, not some abstract view of nursing.

Still on the subject of teaching/learning, Ruddock (1972) points out that a model is developed and refined by an individual. He suggests that the individual's perception, temperament and disposition will influence the kind of ideas and ways of thinking used and the nature of the model which evolves. Ruddock goes on to say that the model may therefore only be understood by individuals of a similar disposition and temperament. It is important that nurses recognise this as a possible limitation, since in nursing not only cognitive structures and processes play a part, but also value systems. This point is further addressed by Webb (1986) when the notions of 'real' and 'soft' science are explored.

Eclecticism

I have addressed the subject of eclecticism elsewhere (Collister, 1986). Eclecticism here refers to a process whereby nurses working in a particular situation may, in an attempt to structure their practice, select elements from different models to fit their reality. Nurses were encouraged to proceed with caution since there was a danger that bits from different models may not fit together. This would be the case especially if different models reflected different value systems, and if these value systems were incompatible each with the other.

At this point I want to take the discussion on this kind of eclecticism a stage further. It has been suggested that each model is, in a sense, idiothetic, since it is a particular instance of how one person conceptualises the phenomenon 'nursing'. Models all represent the same thing and, despite different theoretical perspectives, temperaments and dispositions, there appear to be commonalities between the various models of nursing.

Any nomothetic metaparadigm of nursing, therefore, would subsume all existing models of nursing. This would suggest that rather than selecting elements from different models nurses should select first one model, then a second, integrating this with the first, and so on, gradually building up a model which incorporates all the concepts relative to nursing practice in whatever setting.

Such an approach incorporating not only models of nursing but also models of therapeutic care is displayed by several contributors to this book.

It could be that a metaparadigm of nursing would include all models of nursing currently in existence, all those yet to be developed and published, and all other theory which provides knowledge for nurses in practice.

Some concluding remarks

I have addressed two main themes in this discussion. The first was the metaphorical nature of nursing models which should help nurses to understand, analyse and develop nursing practice. The metaphor suggests that nursing is 'like' something, not that nursing 'is' something. Any attempts to apply the metaphor too rigidly, without challenge, may serve no purpose. What is needed is, as Roper (1986) has suggested, a spirit of informed criticism, not uncritical acceptance.

The second theme in this introduction sought to emphasise the intermediate role that nursing models play between, for example, a care plan for one patient at one point in time and a 'general theory of nursing goals, action and evaluation criteria'.

Mention was made of the way in which nursing models appear to have been integrated into curricula for basic and in-service education. It behoves nurse educators and managers, at whatever level, and in whatever relationship to the organisation, to bear in mind a few simple ideas when asking (or telling) practitioners to use a particular model.

1 Make sure *you* understand the model before asking someone else to take it on. In particular, remember that it is not theory which is being applied, but knowledge, through the performance of skills. Do *you* know what knowledge and can *you* perform the skills?
2 Recognise the difficulties which others may have in understanding the knowledge and developing the appropriate skills.
3 Anticipate the effects of these difficulties and take remedial action.
4 If you do not understand the model or do not possess the appropriate skills, are unable to teach or advise from your own experience, or if you are unable to work through difficulties with others, learning as you go, then have you any right to expect them to do it?
5 If, through refinement, development and discussion a new model seems to be emerging then develop it. (Such an approach is apparent in at least one chapter in this book.)
6 It is essential that the goal of service and the continuing education of practitioners are in harmony. This harmony is achieved through collaborative effort. Teachers and managers therefore need a mutually acceptable and complementary approach, reflected in an appropriate model of practice.

I shall conclude by quoting from the introduction to the first book in this series:

Practising nurses themselves ... must evaluate nursing models and their usefulness in patient care. This process will involve examining what is written about the models, assessing what the models say, and making judgements about their potential contribution to raising the quality of care, enhancing students' learning, and adding to the professional and intellectual standing of nursing.

(Webb, 1986)

It is hoped that this volume will contribute to the process of evaluating the use of models in psychiatric nursing practice.

References

Aggleton P & Chalmers H 1984 I Defining the terms. *Nursing Times*, **80**, 36: 24–28.

Bleuler E 1911 *Dementia Praecox or the Group of Schizophrenias*. (Translated 1951 J Zinkin). Allen & Unwin, London.

Brown GW, Birley JLT & Wing JK 1972 Influence of family life on the course of schizophrenic disorders: A replication. *British Journal of Psychiatry*, **121**: 241–258.

Collister B 1986 Psychiatric nursing and a development model. In *Models for Nursing*, B Kershaw & J Savage (Eds). John Wiley & Sons, Chichester.

Dickoff J & James P 1968 A theory of theories: A position paper. *Nursing Research*, **17**, 3: 197.

Fawcett J 1984 *Analysis and Evaluation of Conceptual Models of Nursing*. FA Davis, Philadelphia.

Freidson E 1970 *The Profession of Medicine*. Dodd, Mead & Co, New York.

Hargie O & McCartan PJ 1986 *Social Skills Training and Psychiatric Nursing*. John Wiley & Sons, Chichester.

Hoenig J & Hamilton MW 1966 The schizophrenic patient under new management. *Comparative Psychiatry*, **7**: 81–91.

Johnson DE 1980 The Behavioural System model for nursing. In *Conceptual Models for Nursing Practice*, J Riehl & C Roy (Eds). Appleton-Century-Crofts, New York.

King IM 1985 A theory for nursing. Paper presented at *Nurse Theorist Conference*, Pittsburgh, 16th May 1985.

Kluckhohn C & Murray HA 1949 *Personality in Nature, Society and Culture*. Cape, London.

Kraepelin E 1906 *Lectures on Clinical Psychiatry*, 2nd Ed. Bailliere Tindall, London.

Orem DE 1980 *Nursing: Concepts of Practice*, 2nd Ed. McGraw-Hill Book Co, New York.

Rogers C 1978 *Carl Rogers on Personal Power*. Constable, London.

Roper N 1986 Developing a model for nursing and relating it to practice. Paper presented at *Models of Nursing Conference*, Eastbourne, 22nd October 1986.

Roy C 1980 The Roy Adaptation model. In *Conceptual Models for Nursing Practice*, J Riehl & C Roy (Eds). Appleton-Century-Crofts, New York.

Ruddock R 1972 *Six Approaches to the Person*. Routledge & Kegan Paul, London.

Scheff TJ 1967 *Mental Illness and Social Processes*. Harper & Row, New York.

Sim M 1981 *Guide to Psychiatry*, 4th Ed. Churchill Livingstone, Edinburgh.

Simon W, Wirt AL, Wirt RD & Halloran A 1965 Long-term follow-up study of schizophrenic patients. *Archives of General Psychiatry*, **12**: 510–515.

Strauss A, Schatzman L, Bucher R, Ehrlich D & Sabshin M 1964 *Psychiatric Ideologies and Institutions*. Free Press, Glencoe, Illinois.

Szasz T 1960 The Myth of Mental Illness. *American Psychologist*, **15**: 113–118.

Webb C (Ed) 1986 *Women's Health. Midwifery and Gynaecological Nursing*. Hodder & Stoughton, Sevenoaks.

2

Care plan for a withdrawn person, based on Orlando's Psychodynamic model

Ben Thomas

There is an absence of published research into the nursing care of the withdrawn individual. This chapter identifies this lack and, it is suggested, serves as a case study of the nursing care of a withdrawn individual. It uses the principles of Orlando's (1961) model to guide nursing action and in doing so demonstrates how the nursing intervention constituted deliberative action rather than *ad hoc* responses.

No argument is made for the use of the model in all nursing situations but it is suggested that the model is of practical value and is well suited to the reality of nursing a person presenting with a problem of withdrawal.

The problem of withdrawal

The term 'withdrawn' is widely used within psychiatric nursing circles, and for the most part its meaning is taken for granted. Withdrawal behaviour may be expressed physically and/or psychologically. We have probably all expressed some form of withdrawal behaviour at some time or another, probably reacting in a constructive way by removing ourselves from a source of danger or threat. However, this type of reaction may also be destructive, leading to social isolation and interfering with normal living activities. It is in this second context that withdrawal is identified as a problem for the individual, and sometimes becomes the concern of psychiatric nurses.

Despite the common usage of the term, there appear to be few published reports of investigations into the problem of withdrawal. The few reports that are in existence usually describe the effect of social isolation experienced by long-term patients in various institutions, for example, Carter and Galliano (1981).

The lack or research into the area of the more acutely withdrawn person has left psychiatric nurses with few guidelines for caring for such persons. What is available to guide the practice of psychiatric nursing in this area has either been borrowed from other disciplines or is based on tradition. Whilst agreeing with Darcy (1980) that psychiatric nursing theory should be built up from practice, it is proposed that practising psychiatric nurses need some practical framework to assist them in caring for the patients they encounter and the problems that these patients may present with, and the day-to-day interactions they have with such patients. It is with these issues in mind that an appropriate nursing model was sought and utilised in caring for a withdrawn patient. In examining the diversity of nursing models that are now in existence it was not intended naively to seek a straightforward, usable solution and then to advocate its adoption into a rigid procedural approach. Rather, the intention has been to select a useful model that could be integrated into a flexible and creative approach in the reality of nursing practice.

Choice of model

The rationale for the choice of Orlando's model is based on the premise that it is now widely recognised that the interpersonal relationship between the nurse and the patient is central to the practice of psychiatric nursing, as suggested by Robinson (1983) and Stuart and Sundeen (1983). Orlando's model of the dynamic nurse–patient relationship incorporates this philosophy, and emphasises the importance of the interaction that occurs between the nurse and the patient.

Stuart and Sundeen (1983) suggest that in the case of a withdrawn patient, the nurse's task of establishing and maintaining a therapeutic relationship is even more complicated than it is with other patients. Any nurse who has experienced trying to communicate with a withdrawn patient is well aware of the frustrations and the uncomfortable feelings that are sometimes aroused in such a situation. The step-by-step description offered by Orlando guides the nurse at various stages of the interaction and ensures that the nurse constantly explores her reaction to the patient and tries to understand what is happening between herself and the patient. Orlando's model then, with its focus on the nurse–patient relationship and the interaction that goes on between them provides a framework for the psychiatric nurse to establish a relationship with a withdrawn patient in a purposeful way.

Outline and critique of the model

It is not my intention to present a complete analysis of Orlando's model as this is well documented elsewhere, for example Andrews (1983) and Crane (1985). However, in order to give those readers who may be unfamiliar with Orlando's work some understanding I shall briefly outline the model by discussing it under the four concepts which are generally agreed to constitute the nursing paradigm (Chinn and Jacobs, 1983). Andrews (1983) argues that although Orlando does not fully develop or refine the concepts of person, health, or environment, she does perceive these concepts as properties characteristic of nursing and defines them within the framework of her model of nursing. Andrews suggests therefore, that their meanings

are understood within the framework of Orlando's nursing model.

Person

According to Orlando a person is defined as a 'behaving human organism'. However, because nursing as a profession has traditionally aligned itself with the practice of medicine, Orlando suggests that nursing knowledge and nursing practice deal only with persons who are under medical supervision or treatment. (I will return to this issue later in considering the major criticisms of the Orlando model.) Orlando does however, draw a sharp distinction between nursing and medicine. She defines medicine as being concerned with the prevention and treatment of disease. Professional nursing on the other hand aims to supply whatever help a patient requires in order for their needs to be met. Nursing is concerned with providing direct assistance to individuals in whatever setting for the purpose of avoiding, relieving, and diminishing the individual's sense of helplessness. Orlando points out that the nurse must learn to understand patients and their needs because those needs that individuals can meet on their own are not of professional concern to the nurse. It is important then that the nurse recognises the individuality of the person, and the consequent unique situations. Crane (1985) suggests that this focus on a patient as a unique individual means that appropriate nursing actions for two patients, even with the same presenting behaviour, must be individualised. The nurse cannot automatically act on principles, past experience, or doctor's orders.

Environment

The environment is important for Orlando because it affects the immediate and individual character of a nursing situation. The nurse must work with the patient in a specific time and place and what the nurse observes, and how the nurse acts are strongly related to the context. Orlando also points out that the environment can cause an unmet need to occur so that nursing action may consist of changing the immediate environment.

Health

While health is not specified in Orlando's writings, it is implied. Orlando proposes that the nurse achieves her purpose when she contributes to the mental and physical health of the patient. By assisting patients to cope with their sense of helplessness she implies that the nurse contributes to their sense of adequacy and well-being. Andrews (1983) suggests that Orlando interchanges the word health with the word comfort, that is mental and physical comfort. It appears then, that Orlando's concept of health deals with comfort, adequacy and well-being.

Nursing

Nursing for Orlando is unique and independent in its concern for an individual's need for help in an immediate situation. In order to meet this need the nurse must act in a disciplined manner that requires proper training. According to Orlando the purpose of professional nursing is to supply the help a patient requires in order for his needs to be met. Inherent in this definition is what Orlando terms the 'rudimentary concept of nursing', namely

any individual nurses another when he carries, whole or in part, the burden of responsibility for what the person cannot yet, or can no longer do alone.

Orlando suggests that the responsibility of a nurse is to help patients meet their needs. A person who is ill is likely to have his sense of adequacy or well-being disrupted, and the nurse helps the patient maintain or retain his sense of adequacy or well-being in stressful situations associated with the patient's illness. The distress may stem from physical limitations, adverse reactions to the setting, and experiences which prevent the patient from communicating his needs. By identifying the nature of the patient's distress and the need for help the nurse realises her professional function as she provides for the patient's mental and physical comfort, while he is undergoing some form of medical treatment and supervision.

The nurse may help meet the patient's need directly or indirectly; indirectly when she helps the patient obtain the services of a person, agency or resource by which his need can be met, and directly by her own activity in a nursing situation. A nursing situation involves the behaviour of the patient, the reaction of the nurse, and the nursing actions designed for the patient's benefit.

The nurse must first of all initiate a process of helping the patient express the specific meaning of his behaviour in order to understand his distress. Orlando explains that this aspect of nursing practice is particularly important because, 'people are ambivalent in relation to their dependency needs'. The nurse must help the patient explore the distress in order to ascertain the help required to relieve it.

Once the need has been ascertained the nurse acts either 'automatically' or 'deliberatively'. Automatic actions are those carried out for reasons other than resolving an immediate need, that is activities carried out without exploration of the patient's need or consideration of how the nursing activity affects the patient. Examples include routines of patient care, carrying out medical orders and routines which protect the organisation. While it may be evident that routines of care and carrying out medical orders are based on health principles which are intended to help the patient, Orlando suggests that deliberation is needed to determine whether the activity achieves its purpose and whether the patient is helped by it.

A deliberative nursing action is clearly related to the nurse's professional function of helping the patient: it involves continuous reflection as the nurse tries to understand the meaning of the patient's behaviour and the action which achieves the purpose of helping the patient. Understanding how practices help or do not help the patient is the material out of which the nurse develops and improves her knowledge and skill in practice.

Criticisms of Orlando's model

As stated earlier it is not intended to present a complete analysis or evaluation of Orlando's model, however, there are three major criticisms of the model which seem worthy of note. The first of these is Orlando's definition of a patient as someone undergoing some form of medical supervision or treatment. This definition has been criticised as being restricted by the consideration of medicine. As Andrews (1983) explains, Orlando's definition of the patient stems from the position of nursing in relation to medicine at the time of Orlando's writing. Andrews suggests that this definition ties nurses and nursing to medical systems and institutions, and therefore restricts the scope of persons, health and environments that may be the concern of nursing. Andrews believes that this reliance upon the medical relationship can be considered a limitation on nursing practice.

The second major criticism concerns Orlando's assumption that nursing interaction is always regarded as immediately beneficial and does not further add to the distress of the patient. This of course may not always be the case, as any nurse who has given a patient an injection or restrained a patient for reasons of safety is well aware. In such circumstances there is usually an increase in distress before a decrease in distress occurs.

Lastly, there is a lack of the social element in Orlando's model. Crane (1985) suggests that Orlando deals only with the interaction between a nurse and a patient in an immediate situation, and does not discuss how the patient is affected by the society in which he lives. Crane argues that the patient should be viewed as a member of a family and within a community for it is often vital to deal with the family as a whole in order to help the patient.

Case history

The following example demonstrates the applicability of Orlando's model to nursing practice. Mary Jones is a 49-year-old married woman with two grown-up children. Mary has lived all her life in the north-west of England. Mary gave up her job in a friend's dress shop in February 1986 because she continually experienced fearfulness and worry about meeting and serving customers. She felt guilty about not working since her income was needed to help support her husband and herself.

Her husband, Jim, had become unemployed in March 1984. Jim had been a building supervisor, but the company he was with went bankrupt and he has not been able to find suitable employment since. Mary's daughter Susan is a hairdresser, but Mary does not see her often as she disapproves of Susan living with her boyfriend. Nor does she see her son John frequently since he moved to London in September 1985 to train as a hotel manager.

Mary was admitted to a general psychiatric ward on 4th March, 1986. During the three months before admission she had experienced fearfulness and worry in any social setting. This had resulted in her isolating herself from her family and friends. She spent most of her time sitting around the house, not taking any interest in herself or her surroundings.

On admission Mary appeared to have no motivation to move or talk and confined herself to her room, refusing to mix with other patients or the staff. Although neatly dressed, Mary looked pale and wore no make-up. Her reddened eyes and saddened look signified her desire to be left alone.

Assessment according to Orlando's model

Orlando's assessment phase is set in motion by patient behaviour. Figure 2.1 shows the nurse's assessment of Mary on their first meeting. All patient behaviour, no matter how insignificant, must be considered as an expression of need for help until its meaning to a particular patient in an immediate situation is understood. When a patient experiences a need that cannot be resolved a sense of helplessness occurs and the patient's behaviour reflects this distress. Orlando explains that feelings of helplessness may be due to physical limitations, adverse reactions to the setting or from an inability to communicate effectively. In Mary's case any one of these causes may have been responsible for her presenting behaviour of withdrawal.

Both verbal and non-verbal patient behaviours are important according to Orlando's assessment. The nurse assigned to Mary's care realised the importance of assessing Mary's non-verbal behaviour since Mary was initially unwilling to state

Fig. 2.1 First assessment of patient

Patient's presenting behaviour	Nurse's perception	Nursing action	Patient's reaction
(i) Mary sitting in her room. She lowered her eyes as I approached her and turned her back towards me.	Mary appears tense and uncomfortable.	(i) I said 'Hello, Mary. I am your primary nurse, Susan. Do you mind if I sit down and talk to you?'	Mary made no verbal response. She continued to sit with her back towards me.
	Nurse's thought: Mary looks upset and does not want me around.	(ii) I said 'I feel rather awkward that you are not looking at me.'	Mary continued to sit in the same position.
	Nurse's feeling: I feel awkward and hurt that Mary does not want to have anything to do with me, but I feel obliged to talk to her.	(iii) I said 'It seems as if you are finding it difficult to say anything right now. I'll leave you for a while and come back at 10 am to see you.'	Mary again made no verbal response and continued to sit in the same position.

how she felt or verbally volunteer any other information. The nurse's close observation of Mary's appearance and non-verbal behaviour indicated Mary's discomfort at the nurse's presence. It also provided a data baseline for future interactions, even though this was not useful to the immediate situation of the patient.

The sharing of the nurse's reaction in Orlando's assessment is a process of exploration with the patient, which allowed the nurse the opportunity to summarise Mary's non-verbal responses.

Problems and goals

Since Orlando deals with the immediate nurse–patient interaction, only one problem is dealt with at a time. Initially the problem of Mary not talking to her primary nurse was identified, as shown in Fig. 2.2. The sharing of the nurse's reaction with Mary revealed that Mary did not talk to her primary nurse because she regarded the nurse as young and inexperienced and therefore questioned her capabilities and skills in being able to help her, as shown in the outcome of the nursing care plan Fig. 2.3.

Orlando's model was particularly useful in this instance because of the interactive process the nurse has to learn in order to understand what is

happening between herself and the patient, and to identify and deal with the feelings of annoyance and hurt which were generated by the continual rejection by Mary. Orlando points out that regardless of the form of the patient's presenting behaviour, for example refusing to speak, the nurse must view it as a possible signal of distress or a manifestation of an unmet need.

According to Orlando's process a goal is always relief of the patient's need for help: any type of goal beyond the immediate situation is not therefore possible. At this stage it could be argued that the nurse's action increased Mary's distress. However, the objective relates to improvement in the patient's behaviour and it could also be argued that an improvement did occur in that Mary's behaviour changed from not talking to giving an explanation of her behaviour. This point will be taken up again when criticisms of the model in use are discussed.

Intervention

Orlando offers a principle to guide the nurse in her reaction to patient behaviour. The nurse does not assume that any aspect of her reaction to the patient is correct, helpful or appropriate until she checks the validity of it in exploration with the patient.

Fig. 2.2   Care plan 1

Problem	Goal	Nursing action	Outcome
Mary does not talk to her primary nurse.	Mary will speak to her primary nurse on at least one occasion over the next eight hours.	1 Primary nurse will approach Mary every 2 hours and offer to spend at least 10 minutes with her.	1 The primary nurse approached Mary at 08.00 hrs, 10.00 hrs, and offered to spend at least ten minutes with her.
		2 Primary nurse will invite Mary to agree on a time for them to meet together.	2 Mary did not reply verbally.
		3 Primary nurse will observe Mary's verbal and non-verbal behaviour.	3 Mary closed her eyes on the first two occasions. She looked briefly at me on the third. She lay curled up on her bed for the whole morning.
		4 Primary nurse will disclose to Mary her understanding of the interaction.	4 I said to Mary that she looked very sad, and that I felt uncomfortable about not being able to help her.

Orlando terms this a deliberative nursing process, which involves continuous reflection as the nurse tries to understand the meaning of the behaviour to the patient.

It was evident that Mary did not respond quickly to the nursing intervention and the process of reflection enabled the nurse to assess the level of necessary intervention which at the beginning consisted of offering to spend a small, consistent amount of time with the patient. The length of time was decided both by Mary and the nurse, and at first much of this time was spent in silence. Barker (1985) argues that silences should be avoided when dealing with a passive and withdrawn patient, and that it is now generally accepted that the nurse should become more active to compensate for this. However, Stuart and Sundeen (1983) suggest that constant chatter may convey to the patient the message that there is no expectation for her to verbalise. Since the goal of the nursing intervention was for Mary to talk to her primary nurse, then the primary nurse had to provide the opportunity for this to occur. By approaching Mary every two hours and inviting her to agree on a time for them to meet, the primary nurse demonstrated her consistency, reliability and accessibility, and thereby fostered a sense of trust.

Evaluation

Evaluation is inherent in Orlando's action phase of her deliberative process. For an action to be deliberative the nurse must evaluate its effectiveness when it is completed. The nurse observed Mary's behaviour to see whether she had been helped. In the first instance this involved observing Mary's non-verbal cues such as eye contact and body posture.

The consistent repeated approaches by the nurse were aimed at convincing Mary of the nurse's sincere interest and concern for her and the establishing of a nurse–patient relationship. When Mary stated that she was unwilling to talk to the primary nurse because of her youth and inexperi-

Fig. 2.3   Care plan 2

Problem	Goal	Nursing action	Outcome
Mary does not talk to her primary nurse.	Mary will speak to her primary nurse on at least one occasion over the next eight hours.	1 Primary nurse will approach Mary every 2 hours and offer to spend at least 10 minutes with her.	1 The primary nurse approached Mary at 13.00 hrs and 15.00 hrs and offered to spend 10 minutes with her.
		2 Primary nurse will invite Mary to agree on a time limit for them to meet together.	2 Mary did not reply verbally at 13.00 hrs but at 15.00 hrs Mary said 'There's no point in me talking to you, you're too young to understand and too inexperienced to help me'.
		3 Primary nurse will observe Mary's verbal and non-verbal behaviour.	3 Mary looked directly at me as I approached at 13.00 hrs but looked out of the window while she spoke to me.
		4 Primary nurse will disclose to Mary her understanding of the interaction.	4 I said to Mary that I heard what she said but that I still wanted to try and help her and I would leave her to think about my offer.

ence, the nurse acknowledged Mary's distress and the focus of the nursing action changed to inviting Mary to join the nurse in an activity of her choosing, as shown in Fig. 2.4. The primary nurse therefore decreased Mary's distress by removing the expectation of Mary to talk to the nurse until Mary felt she was able to do so. This also allowed Mary to control the pace of the development of closeness and disclosure.

The deliberative nursing action resulted in Mary spending designated periods of time with the primary nurse in various activities. During these activities the primary nurse observed Mary's verbal and non-verbal behaviour. These observations provided the nurse with the necessary cues to take further action. For example, when Mary retained constant eye contact with the nurse and relaxed her previously tense body posture this demonstrated an increased comfort with the nurse. The nurse's reaction was to feel more at ease. The nurse verbally expressed her reaction to Mary by stating, 'You appear to be more relaxed with me now, Mary, which makes me feel more comfortable.' The nurse not only gave Mary an opportunity then to know what her reaction was but she also gave her the opportunity to correct or validate her reaction. As Mary and the nurse began to relate more comfortably, other nurses and patients were gradually included in Mary's social sphere. At first this was a problem for Mary as shown in Fig. 2.5. However, by inviting other patients and nurses to join in activities with Mary, and helping Mary relate to them, Mary was eventually able to develop interpersonal relationships with a variety of people.

Fig. 2.4   Care plan 3

Problem	Goal	Nursing action	Outcome
Mary does not talk to her primary nurse because she thinks the nurse is young and inexperienced and therefore unable to help her.	Mary will join with her primary nurse in an activity of Mary's choice for at least 10 minutes over the next eight hours.	1 Primary nurse will approach Mary at the beginning of the shift and arrange a time for Mary to join with her for at least 10 minutes.	1 Primary nurse approached Mary at the beginning of the shift and arranged to meet Mary at 10.30 hrs to walk with her to the hospital shop to buy a packet of cigarettes.
		2 Primary nurse will observe Mary's verbal and non-verbal behaviour.	2 Mary stated that the only thing she wanted to do was to buy some cigarettes. She maintained steady eye contact with me during the time she spoke.
		3 Primary nurse will meet Mary at the agreed time and engage with Mary in the selected activity.	3 Met Mary at 10.30 hrs and walked with her to the hospital shop and Mary bought a packet of cigarettes.
			4 We walked slowly to the shop and Mary asked me how far we had to walk. On returning to the ward she thanked me for showing her where the shop was.

Critique of the model in use

Since Orlando only deals with immediate nurse–patient interaction, only one need is dealt with at a time and any type of goal beyond the immediate situation is not taken into account. However, while Orlando's process guided the nurse in a series of sequential steps which were effective because the nurse constantly explored her reactions with the patient in the individual situation, the medium through which the improvement occurred, i.e. the establishment of the nurse–patient relationship, could be argued to have an accumulative effect over a period of time. It was also necessary to see Mary's care in terms of setting long-term goals. These

consisted of Mary eventually attending ward group meetings and participating in social activities outside the ward situation.

Another problem is that Orlando regards nursing interaction as always being beneficial and not adding to the distress of the patient. As previously discussed this is not always the case. In the initial stages of forming a relationship it was obvious that Mary's distress was increased by the nurse's advances, since all of Mary's behaviour demonstrated that she wanted to be left alone. Even though, through the deliberative nursing action it was established that this was not really the case at the time, an increase in distress did occur before it eventually decreased.

Orlando's model is also limited by its focus on

Fig. 2.5   Care plan 4

Problem	Goal	Nursing action	Outcome
Mary does not socialise with the other patients on the ward.	Mary will join her primary nurse and two other patients on the ward in a game of Scrabble for half an hour over the next eight hours.	1 Primary nurse will approach Mary and invite her to join in a game of Scrabble with 2 other patients and herself for half an hour.	1 Primary nurse approached Mary and invited her to join in a game of Scrabble with 2 other patients and herself for half an hour.
		2 Primary nurse will observe Mary's verbal and non-verbal behaviour.	2 Mary stated that she used to play Scrabble with her children, and although she had not played it for a long time, she was willing to have a go.
		3 Primary nurse will introduce Mary to the other 2 patients and join in a game of Scrabble.	3 Primary nurse introduced Mary to Peter and Carole.
		4 Primary nurse will observe Mary's verbal and non-verbal behaviour.	4 Mary smiled quickly at Peter and Carole but did not speak. About 20 minutes into the game Mary spontaneously asked Carole how long she had been in hospital? When asked questions by Peter and Carole, Mary answered them by speaking quietly and slowly. At the end of the game Mary accepted Carole's offer to join her for a cup of coffee.

interaction with an individual, whereas it has been argued earlier that it may be necessary to view the patient as a member of a family and within a community. The members of Mary's family played an important part in her life and her problem, and it was necessary to deal with the family as a whole in order to help Mary and in the formulation of long-term plans, which as previously discussed, Orlando's model does not cater for.

Management and education implications

The ability to implement Orlando's model in caring for this patient was undoubtedly aided by having a system of primary nursing in operation on the ward. This meant that the same nurse had consistent contact with the patient throughout her stay in hospital and enhanced the effective development of the one-to-one relationship which was deemed necessary for helping the patient. The behaviours learned in this nurse–patient relationship were then transferred to other interpersonal relationships with a variety of other people.

The purpose of Orlando's model of nursing was to offer the student of professional nursing a theory of effective nursing practice. The concepts and propositions in Orlando's model offered clear and relevant guides which were applicable for nursing a patient with a problem of withdrawal. In each contact with the patient the nurse repeated a process of learning how to help that individual patient. As Orlando points out, understanding how practices help or do not help the patient is the material out of which the nurse develops her knowledge and skill in practice and her professional role and identity.

Learning to understand what is happening between oneself and the patient is the central core of the nurse's practice, according to Orlando. In so doing the nurse has to learn and develop self-awareness skills which are now regarded as essential psychiatric nursing skills, as described by the Syllabus of Training for the Professional Register (English National Board, 1982).

References

Andrews CM 1983 Ida Orlando's model of nursing. In *Conceptual Models of Nursing: Analysis and Application*, J Fitzpatrick & A Whall (Eds). Robert J Brady Company, Maryland.

Barker P 1985 *Patient Assessment in Psychiatric Nursing.* Croom Helm, London.

Carter C & Galliano, D 1981 Fear of loss and attachment: A major dynamic in the social isolation of the institutionalized aged. *Journal of Gerontological Nursing*, 7, 6: 342.

Chinn PL & Jacobs MK 1983 *Theory and Nursing: A Systematic Approach.* CV Mosby Co, St Louis.

Crane MD 1985 Ida Jean Orlando. In *Nursing Theories, the Base for Professional Nursing Practice*, JB George (Ed). Prentice-Hall, Englewood Cliffs, New Jersey.

Darcy PT 1980 The nursing process – a base for all nursing developments. *Nursing Times*, **76**, 12: 497–501.

English National Board 1982 *Syllabus of Training, Professional Register: Part 3 (Registered Mental Nurse).* English and Welsh National Boards for Nursing, Midwifery and Health Visiting.

Orlando IJ 1961 *The Dynamic Nurse–Patient Relationship: Function, Process and Principles.* GP Putnam's Sons, New York.

Robinson L 1983 *Psychiatric Nursing as a Human Experience*, 3rd Ed. WB Saunders Co, Philadelphia.

Stuart GW & Sundeen SJ 1983 *Principles and Practice of Psychiatric Nursing*, 2nd Ed. CV Mosby Co, St Louis.

3

Care plan for an agoraphobic person, using an enhancement model of nursing

Felicity Stockwell

This chapter serves as an example of a process identified in Chapter 1 of this book. Stockwell (1985) is in the process of developing a model based on a particular view of nursing. Rather than focusing on patient problems, the enhancement model requires the nurse to identify the patient's strengths and assets and to help the patient capitalise on these in order to overcome problems. It is in this sense that *enhancement* takes place.

This chapter describes the application of the enhancement model in the care of Jean Cox who suffers from agoraphobia. The care is carried out by a Community Psychiatric Nurse.

Phobic states

Phobic states are recognised as being common in western culture, but there is a paucity of research into the aetiology, treatment and prognosis.

The International Classification of Diseases produced by The World Health Organization has a single listing of phobic state at 300.2, but there is general agreement in current literature that it is useful to distinguish between single-symptom phobias and more generalised states of fearfulness such as agoraphobia. The American *Diagnosis and Statistical Manual of Mental Disorder* (1980) divides the phobic neurosis category into four separate categories, one of which is agoraphobia with panic attacks.

Agoraphobia is distinguished from anxiety states, with or without panic attacks, by the persistence of the fearfulness, the expression of feelings of either impending disaster or loss of control in specific situations and by the development of avoidance strategies. Medical studies have explored genetic factors in agoraphobia (e.g., Crowe *et al.*, 1983), alcohol dependence (e.g., Smail, 1984), and Michelson *et al.* (1986) describe a study that compared the effect of four different treatment strategies. Follow-up studies have been carried out on psychotherapy and behavioural programmes and some studies have explored personality factors and the personality and involvement of the spouse (e.g., Barlow *et al.*, 1984).

Nursing texts suggest that the nurse's role in caring for patients with agoraphobia can be to educate the patient in relaxation techniques (e.g., Lyttle, 1986); to provide support and care and opportunity to experiment with more useful patterns of behaviour until treatment is effective (e.g., Irving, 1983); and, where relevant, to supervise and encourage the patient's participation in a behavioural programme (e.g., Dexter and Wash, 1986). Paykel and Griffith (1983) showed that nurses could be given a large amount of autonomy within the multidisciplinary team to provide therapeutic nursing for neurotic patients in the community, and the patients in the study did not express any dissatisfaction at having less contact with the psychiatrist.

In some instances nurses are trained to plan and implement behavioural therapy as therapists in their own right and, as detailed in Marks *et al.* (1977), agoraphobia has been shown to be a suitable diagnostic category for such therapists. However, this chapter will only concern itself with nursing in the traditional role where the doctor retains the responsibility for the patient while the nurse carries out the treatment that has either been particularly prescribed or is within the context of the team's philosophy and practice.

Outline and critique of an enhancement model of nursing

The enhancement model perceives the patient as a unique being who is always more than the sum of the parts, however comprehensively these may be defined or listed.

This unique being becomes a patient who needs nursing, either because pathology interferes with his ability to manage life, or stresses and conflict prevent a healthy life-style to a degree that requires some help and support from others.

The nurse is seen as a skilled interactor and knowledgeable carer who has a human and professional interest in the welfare of the patient. It is this welfare that is the prime responsibility of nursing and while the safety of the patient has to have priority this model suggests that by focusing on the patient's strengths and abilities and planning and implementing strategies to enhance them, nursing could provide the potential for the patient's experience of mental illness to contribute positively and beneficially to their life experience.

Both patient and nurse have many innate and learned capabilities, skills and aptitudes and have been subject to a large range of influences and experiences, and when they meet at a point on their journeys through life these will determine the content and quality of the interaction, and whatever happens between them will become part of their futures.

Figure 3.1 shows the separate life paths of the patient and the nurse but gives them the same emphasis and puts them at the same level to indicate that, in terms of experience and value, both can contribute equally to the relationship.

With regard to the activities of nursing, the model reflects the fact that, at the time of implementation, psychiatric nursing is nearly always a personal activity between one nurse and one patient. This holds true for group activities because unless the nurse has rapport with each individual member of the group they will not benefit. However, it also recognises that nursing is usually a team endeavour and so the philosophy of the nursing process, with its systematic and shared approach to assessing, planning, implementing and evaluating nursing care, has been incorporated. The commitment to identifying and enhancing strengths as a primary concern can be embraced by the team as well as by individuals.

Although this model focuses on nursing at an interpersonal level, with the prime responsibility being to ensure the patient's welfare, it recognises that many other people, both professional and lay, contribute to the patient's progress and well-being. Hopefully, it should be possible to share the enhancement philosophy with these others.

Nurses have a repertoire of skilled interventions to minimise difficulties and disabilities that may be evident or troubling the patient. These certainly form an important part of nursing and this is given recognition in the model but again, these remedies can be more effective when they build on or utilise the patient's strengths.

The model purposefully avoids the identification of problems as the focus of attention for several reasons. Firstly, an interview that explores all the negatives can leave the patient feeling interesting but bleak; then, having identified problems, there is the possibility that some or many of them are not within the nurse's power to solve. Also, it is likely that when planning care and sharing the resources, the patients with many or unusual problems will receive extra attention.

So the enhancement model of nursing embraces the realities of nursing while exploiting the potential of the patient's experience of being mentally ill to provide a rewarding and positive contribution to his life pattern, and it sees the nurse's various skills as playing an important part in helping to achieve this, while, through learning, she also gains from the experience.

A criticism of this model is that because a person can have strengths and abilities in every facet of his

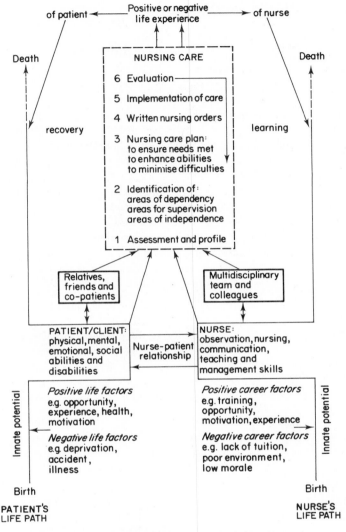

Fig. 3.1 An enhancement model of psychiatric nursing

functioning there is no construct to provide a framework for assessing and planning care. For the experienced nurse this can be an asset because it leaves her free to focus on whatever relevant strengths the patient demonstrates, exploring leads that are likely to be useful, while recognising what nursing strategies are going to be needed. For the beginner, guidelines to all the areas of capability can be provided. These can be grouped under physical, intellectual, emotional, social and spiritual headings and should be referred to before and after the interview but not during it. With good questioning and listening skills the interview should leave the patient feeling he has shared all he wants to, has highlighted the help he needs and has left a good impression, and not feeling, as can be the case in some admission procedures, as if he has been interrogated for the benefit of the staff and the records.

A case study of agoraphobia

Jean Cox is a 27-year-old woman who is a qualified librarian, married to a design engineer.

She has been married for five years and had intended to continue working after her son was born two years ago, as her family was willing to share in his care. However, her husband's job required him to move across the country just four months after the baby's birth, so she decided not to seek work as they felt the husband's rise in salary would enable them to manage financially and they did not want to leave their son with strangers.

Two weeks ago Jean's husband took her to see her general practitioner because six months earlier she had been convinced she was having a heart attack while visiting the local library and later, while in the supermarket, she had an episode of feeling trapped and panicky. Since then she had become increasingly reluctant to leave the house on her own.

Her husband had tried to help by doing the shopping and accompanying her on outings but she was now phoning him at work with various excuses to get him home during the day. This was causing problems with his employers and in spite of his care his wife's difficulties were getting worse.

When the practice doctor suggested an appointment with a psychiatrist at the local hospital Jean adamantly refused, saying that she could not get there on her own and she would not ask her husband to take her. Because of the difficulties with transport and the nature of her illness she agreed to be referred to the community psychiatric team.

Nursing management based on the enhancement model

Assessment

The community psychiatric nurse (CPN) is making a first visit with the information contained in the case study.

The rationale for using the enhancement model in the assessment of the patient is based on one of the principles of perception (set) where, out of a complex pattern of stimuli certain patterns of cues become the foreground and the focus of attention, while the rest become background and are not given attention. The set of the individual plays a large part in what becomes foreground and where a nurse is concerned with identifying signs and symptoms and problems, then observations and questions will concentrate on these areas, while the patient's strengths and abilities tend to become background and are ignored. If the enhancement model is influencing the nurse it adjusts her set to focus first of all on the well aspects of the person as foreground, encouraging rapport to be established, and then, because the nature of the interaction is to be concerned with any difficulties, these will be attended to and assessed.

The initial frames of reference for observations and exploration will be the areas where Jean is observably functioning or managing to some degree. These could be:

1   Her social interaction and ability to communicate.
2   Her care for, and her relationship with, her son.
3   Her relationship with her husband.
4   Her present life-style and past history, leading on to her present difficulties.
5   Her physiological state of arousal or tension.

Basing the assessment on the enhancement model the CPN will take each frame of reference and for each one will notice all Jean's abilities and competencies and then will formulate questions that put the initial focus on what Jean can manage and enjoy, gradually leading to the areas where she needs help.

Thus the CPN will be aware that Jean is courteous, can chat informally and can make her feel welcome. She may notice that she sits back in her chair with a friendly expression, but has one leg twisted tightly around the other.

She sees that Jean's son looks well cared for and appears to be a lively, normal two-year-old.

She takes in the ambience of the room, notices all the well-read books on the shelf and the television and hi-fi equipment.

Because the enhancement model puts the accent on abilities and strengths the CPN will start her exploration by asking Jean questions about her hobbies and interests and any pleasures she takes in doing things about the house, and will then move on to investigate what social contacts she has, apart from her husband and son.

In this instance Jean replies that the only person she speaks to is the milkman when he calls for the money, but her face lights up as she recounts how he makes her laugh and she uses all sorts of ploys to keep him chatting for a bit longer. The CPN uses the incident to make a joke about housewives and milkmen and they share in laughter, improving rapport and revealing that Jean has a sense of humour.

The lightened atmosphere and Jean's more relaxed stance give the CPN the opportunity to start investigating her difficulties, but still the questioning begins by putting the accent on the things she can do. Jean has said that she can't go out anywhere on her own but admits to going to the dustbin and the washing line. When asked if she could manage to go to the end of the road on her own she replies that she doesn't know. At this point the CPN suggests that she might like to try it, either on her own or with her son – just to the end of the road and straight back, noticing all the while what she is feeling, so she can share it when she returns. Providing this suggestion is based on sound observation and evaluation Jean will probably agree and manage quite comfortably. In which case the CPN has gained some factual observations, has generated some shared experience and laid the foundation for the nursing programme.

This first session ends with discussion and agreement about what they hope to achieve together and the setting of some preliminary objectives, and an appointment for the next session.

Planning

Both Jean and the CPN hope that the outcome of their work together will be that Jean will be able to get out and about without any apprehension.

The first decision that has to be made is whether to visit Jean in her own home or to see her at the day hospital. Gournay (1986) found no difference in outcome in patients with agoraphobia treated at home or attending a day hospital, so, providing there are no constraints of time or cost this offers an open choice. All nursing involves choices of action (or inaction) and a decision about how, when and where to carry them out. Each individual nurse's philosophy will influence her choices and decisions and it is in this area that the statements of a model have their major effect.

This particular choice can be used to illustrate how viewpoints of different models can influence a nurse's decisions and interaction with a patient.

A model that sees nursing as meeting unmet needs falls easily into a problem-solving approach to planning care. In this instance the problem is that the patient cannot get out and travel to the day hospital on her own, and this means that her social and communication needs are not being met. The rational solution to this problem is to provide transport because that best meets the patient's needs in terms of the problem. Jean might not be able to manage even with transport so it would then be expedient to see her in her own home, but that would be a second best solution that could leave her feeling that she was particularly ill or being a nuisance.

With the enhancement model, the first step is to recognise what strengths Jean has shown in relation to the choice as to where to see her. In this instance it could be that the CPN recognises that Jean has managed to act as a hostess very well, making her feel at ease and welcome, and this could influence her to decide to see her at home to begin with. Or she could use the fact that Jean managed to walk to the end of the road better than she anticipated to explore whether she would like the challenge of visiting the day hospital if transport was provided. Another aspect of the decision is to determine which choice is most likely to offer opportunity for the next step in developing Jean's potential. In this case, because the move has reduced Jean's social contacts in all the areas of her life it is likely that social isolation is the most important factor in precipitating Jean's agoraphobia. It could be argued that to help Jean to invite a neighbour with a toddler in for coffee would be a useful first step towards recovery, though again this has to be weighed against the fact that Jean could experience a rewarding sense of achievement if she could manage to travel to the day hospital, and she might make friends with someone in the waiting room.

If, as in this instance, both choices seem to be

equally enhancing there are other factors that can be weighed in the balance. The nurse should attempt to forecast which course of action is least likely to be detrimental to the patient if the objective is not achieved, and if this does not enable a decision then the choice that requires the most time and effort from the nurse will probably be the most enhancing!

At some point in the planning the CPN is likely to confer with her colleagues and other members of the multidisciplinary team and they will draw up broad objectives that will be more clearly defined in discussion with Jean and her husband. These objectives will probably include:

1   teaching conscious control of tension through relaxation techniques;
2   teaching breath control;
3   outlining a hierarchy of outings;
4   setting up social contacts for Jean;
5   gaining the husband's interest and cooperation.

Implementation

The enhancement model of nursing influences the nurse while she carries out the planned activities by encouraging her to remember that the way in which she interacts with the patient will not only affect the outcome of intervention but will be incorporated into the patient's life experience, to be remembered as either beneficial or detrimental. Hopefully the nurse will be motivated to ensure that the patient's experience of being nursed will be a good one.

The way in which the enhancement model influences the implementation of nursing can be illustrated by looking at the way the CPN involves the health visitor in helping to exercise Jean's social abilities.

In approaching the health visitor the CPN could say, 'I have a client who is agoraphobic. She moved here eighteen months ago and hasn't managed to make any friends and now can't get out at all. I wonder if you have a client who might be willing to call in to see her'. On the other hand with the influence of the enhancement model the CPN could say, 'I have a client who is a very intelligent, pleasant woman, and sociable and friendly until she moved here eighteen months ago. She hasn't made

friends with anyone since she moved and is now finding it very difficult to get out at all. Do you know anyone who might enjoy calling round to see her?'.

Thus the client is presented in a positive light, the intervention is suggested as being potentially rewarding to both parties, and the health visitor is encouraged to think positively in terms of who she approaches.

This philosophy does not preclude encouraging and testing a patient's independence by expressing anger or teasing, providing the patient is resilient enough and an enhancing rapport is well established. The ultimate aim of all nursing is that patients should become confidently independent of the nurse, unless they are terminally ill, in which case skilled care and comfort is the priority.

So, as the nurse establishes a friendly relationship with Jean and builds a bridge of trust between them, Jean will begin to realise she is the determiner of her own recovery and will be given the help, encouragement and motivation to achieve the objectives of the care plan.

Evaluation

With this model of nursing, judging to what extent the nursing has been beneficial has to focus on the patient's self-esteem, their self-respect and their happiness. Beyond this it is then necessary, as in the assessment stage, to check all the frames of reference to ensure that the client is functioning fully in each area, and where there is any residual disability to ensure that it is helped or compensated for as much and as beneficially as possible.

References

Barlow DH, O'Brien GT & Last CG 1984 Couples treatment of agoraphobia. *Behaviour Therapy*, **15**: 41–53.

Burglass D, Clarke J, Henderson AS, Kreitman N & Pressley AS 1977 A study of agoraphobic housewives. *Psychological Medicine*, **7**: 73–86.

Crowe RR, Noyes R, Pauls DL & Slymen D 1983 A family study of psychiatric disorders. *Archives of General Psychiatry*, **40**, 10: 1065–1069.

Dexter G & Wash M 1986 *Psychiatric Nursing Skills.* Croom Helm, London.

Diagnostic and Statistical Manual of Mental Disorder, 3rd Ed. 1980 American Psychiatric Association, Washington DC.

Gelder MG   1986   Panic attacks: New approaches to an old problem. *British Journal of Psychiatry*, **149**, 9: 347.

Gournay D   1986   *Agoraphobia and its behavioural treatment.* Unpublished thesis, University of Leicester. (Author's abstract in *Nursing Research*.)

Harris EL, Noyes R, Crowe RR & Chaudry DR   1983   A family study of agoraphobia. *Archives of General Psychiatry*, **40**: 1061–1064.

Hilgard ER, Atkinson RC & Atkinson RL   1975   *Introduction to Psychology.* Harcourt Brace Jovanovich, New York.

Irving S   1983   *Basic Psychiatric Nursing.* WB Saunders Co, Philadelphia.

Lyttle J   1986   *Mental Disorder.* Bailliere Tindall, London.

Marks IM   1975   *Fears and Phobias.* Heinemann Medical, London.

Marks IM, Hallam RS, Connolly J & Philpott R 1977   *Nursing in Behavioural Psychotherapy.* Royal College of Nursing, London.

Michelson L, Mavissakalion M, Marchione K, Dancu C & Greenwald M   1986   The role of self-directed *in vivo* exposure in cognitive, behavioural and psychosocial treatments of agoraphobia. *Behaviour Therapy*, **17**, 2: 91–110.

Paykel ES & Griffith JH   1983   *Community Psychiatric Nursing for Neurotic Patients.* Royal College of Nursing, London.

Russell GFM & Hersov LA (Eds)   1983   *Handbook of Psychiatry 4.* Cambridge University Press. (pp.218–222).

Smail P, Stockwell T, Canter S & Hodgson R 1984   Alcohol dependence and phobic anxiety states. I. A prevalence study. *British Journal of Psychiatry*, **144**: 53–57.

Stockwell F   1985   *The Nursing Process in Psychiatric Nursing.* Croom Helm, London.

4

Care plan for a man receiving domiciliary care, using Peplau's model of nursing

Bill Lemmer

This chapter is about the therapeutic use of interpersonal relationships. A developmental model of nursing is applied to the care of a middle-aged son living as a 'passive receptor' (Peplau, 1952; p.244) with his mother. Following a brief introduction, the chapter examines assessment, analyses the nursing offered, and reviews the theoretical framework, making reference to the nursing process format for recording and evaluating interpersonal relationships.

My client and I agreed to use his nursing as an example of care for publication. Therefore, certain details are omitted to preserve confidentiality. However, the nature of our agreement enables us to share a detailed example of the Peplau (1952) model of nursing at work.

Editorial comment

Peplau does not see the nursing process as a series of steps involving assessment, planning, implementation and evaluation; her writing pre-dates most of the literature which takes this view of the steps/stages of the nursing process.

Instead, the process she focuses on is the developing relationship between the nurse and the patient, Peplau (1952) describes four phases to this relationship: orientation, identification, exploitation and resolution. These phases are not discrete, and hence a degree of overlap between them may be recognised. Peplau describes the characteristics of these phases and, at any one time, the features of at least two of them may be recognised in an interaction between the nurse and the patient. However, it is also possible to identify the steps of the nursing process in relation to these phases. The overlap between the phases of the nurse–patient relationship, and their links with the nursing process, are represented schematically in Fig. 4.1. Attention is also drawn to the idea, illustrated in Fig. 4.1, that the steps of the nursing process are not themselves discrete, and that evaluation is not a once-and-for-all event but is continuous throughout the cycle.

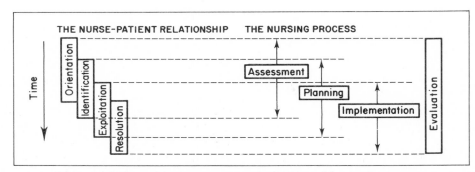

Fig. 4.1 Phases of the nurse–patient relationship and the nursing process

The problem-solving cycle (assessing, planning, implementing and evaluating) occurs frequently during, and between, each encounter with the patient. Assessment and implementation are carried out through the medium of communication (a key concept in Peplau's model) and involve activities by the nurse, feedback from the patient, and vice versa. Planning and evaluation are cognitive activities on the part of the nurse. These latter activities are often not recorded, but the use of process recordings (Peplau, 1952: p.308) means that validation and decision making are a conscious and deliberative effort.

The process recordings included in this chapter show the developing relationship between the nurse and the patient, and the phases are indicated on p.29. In the process recordings it is also possible to identify the stages of the problem-solving cycle. However, these stages would be more obvious through the use of some sort of problem orientated record. Such a record could show:

1   *Problem identification, patient outcomes, intervention and evaluation for each encounter or series of encounters. The goals would be short term and relate to the phases of the developing relationship as well as particular problems.*
2   *A similarly structured overall care plan showing long-term goals for each problem. This would be updated as short- and medium-term goals were achieved.*

This approach is demonstrated in two other chapters in this book, in the care of a withdrawn person (Chapter 2) and an aggressive person (Chapter 10).

Blair Collister

Selection of model

Even though a model of nursing is used, I am aware that the way it is used is influenced by my past experience. There are four main threads to the way I view nursing:

1   My study for the diploma and my nursing practice at the Cassel Hospital, in Surrey. This is a National Health Service therapeutic community, where the care of individuals is community-centred (Barnes, 1968). The values of this nursing are centred upon opening lines of communication, such as the nurse facilitating groups of clients, or working alongside a group preparing a meal, for example, the nurse talking one-to-one with a client, but also being a member of an interdisciplinary team. Teaching at the Cassel is focused upon the nurse's relationships, and I find it interesting that Peplau's model also focuses upon the nurse, to promote growth and development in the client.

2   The Cassel experience was followed by a three-year action research project, at a large mental hospital. This project, called 'The Management of Change', attempted to discover learning difficulties in changing from custodial to individualised patient care. This enquiry used the group process as its principal research method for enabling changes in attitudes and perceptions to occur.

3   A third influence upon my nursing has been my involvement with the Training Group of the Interdisciplinary Association for Mental Health Workers. Members of the Training Group come from the various disciplines working in mental health services, for example nursing, psychology, psychiatry, occupational therapy, social work and teaching. Key issues that are inherent in training events offered by this group include the transition from institution to community-based care, interdisciplinary co-operation, participation in care planning by people who use the mental health services, and the development of new services.

4   The final thread of my experience, which bears upon the way I perceive and use models of nursing, is my study and nursing practice during the four years 1983–1987 – this period covered the Diploma in Nursing and the Diploma in Nursing Education.

Peplau's (1952) model of nursing seems congruent with my view of psychiatric nursing. The values which I derive from my experience, which I would say relate to Peplau's notion of helping clients, are discovery, perceiving, observing, expressing, sharing, learning, growing, and developing. The care plan should be a measure of the extent to which these values are demonstrated as nursing skills. Furthermore, is it clear in the care given that the values and skills one develops are useful?

Assessment

Selection of a client

Tom was referred to me by a community psychiatric nurse. He seemed unable to make progress. CPNs and the social workers were puzzled and concerned that on the one hand he posed no overt problems and on the other his lack of progress was a worry to them. I went to the mental health centre to meet Tom, his CPN, and a social worker. We met weekly for three weeks to discuss how I might help and what help he might require, if any. The mental health centre was a busy, lively, houseful of people, with a number of events taking place each day. It was easy to see how Tom's absence, either from the centre or from the activities there, could go unnoticed. After all, he got on okay; he was no problem. Following permission to view Tom's records, the mental health workers' attitudes became more understandable. The measures of progress were the carers' perceptions of Tom's hygiene, non-attendance at the day centre, non-attendance at activities when he was at the centre, and the absence of psychotic symptoms. There was no description in the available records to substantiate a diagnosis, noted variously as delusions of persecution, subnormal intelligence, paranoid delusions, personality disorder and chronic paranoid schizophrenia. Obviously, a lot had happened over many years and a picture of chronic illness had been established. Overall, I was encouraged in the process of getting to know people at the day centre; Tom was keen for us to be together and I was told by staff that he had talked more than they had ever heard before.

Evaluation and analysis of the assessment

Part of the orientation process was to meet Tom's mother and to obtain permission to nurse Tom in the context of the family home. Arguments between mother and son tended, in my observation, to interrupt his activity, interfere with his goals, and stop what he wanted to do. Examples of this occurred when he was washing with his vest on, wanting the same number of cigarettes a day as his

Fig. 4.2   Biographical information and historical data

'Tom' Crossly is the eldest son of Beatrice and her deceased husband, Herbert, who died following a stroke some years ago. Two brothers and a sister live in the vicinity of the family home. Tom, 46, has always lived with his now 70-year-old mother. Together they share the council house where all the children were raised, except Mason. He, Tom, and mother were 'caught' in an air raid during World War II. The intensity of our meetings at their house suggest why a person-centred or developmental picture of the family was difficult to acquire. Details about Mason, for example, were sketchy and inconsistent. However, it seemed that Tom was unmarked, his mother was rescued and hospitalised, and Mason was dead at the scene. The family's appreciation of the past appeared to be lost in the heat of their need to express themselves to me.

Tom is a short, thin man who was described by a consultant psychiatrist as a person who remains well and has not been sick for years. Tom became a user of psychiatric services at the age of 31, when, after an argument with mother, he exchanged blows with her. He was last employed in work at age 30, when for three years he was a council labourer. Prior to that, he worked in odd-jobs, as a cleaner for several years and as a deliveryman's assistant before that. He was admitted 'informally' and, while there is no available record of the length of this hospital admission, it appears from the family that this was for a few months. This was followed by a second admission of less than a month, which also resulted from an argument with mother, with punches being thrown. At the time of the first admission, the mother's daughter was living at home with her infant daughter. Tom's mother said she fed this girl, and the girl called her mother until she and her daughter agreed that the girl should be told not to – by that time the girl was a teenager. Tom's mother's mothering role is a key feature in the collaborative assessment, because it indicated to me and became evident in the family that she was using this role to avoid issues in her own ageing development.

brother, or going for walks instead of going to the mental health centre. This interrupting of his goal-directed activity became evident to Tom during our meetings with mother present (see Fig. 4.3).

The assessment was on two levels, one developmental (Fig. 4.3, encounter 2), and the other practical, i.e. what did he want help with? 'Everything' was his first response. The very activities which Tom found most satisfying were the ones with which his mother seemed to take issue, and he objected to his enjoyment being spoiled.

As I tried to orientate myself, I drew upon the guidelines of Peplau's four psychological tasks:

1   learn to count on others;
2   delay satisfaction;
3   identify oneself;
4   develop skills in participation.

These are the tasks of the client; they demonstrate the extent to which Peplau draws upon developmental psychology. For example, the child as an infant does not know the difference between himself and others. The child learns to differentiate himself from others and develops an identity. Tom's mother disagreed with his spontaneous activity. She also criticised tasks she had agreed with, for example his washing out the milk bottles, or emptying the rubbish. There were always conditions, i.e. emptying the rubbish immediately after having fish and chips because of the smell. Peplau predicted that blocking or interfering with pathways to satisfaction causes frustration, conflict, anxiety, and eventually outrage. Her concept of assessment occurs during a period of orientation:

> To encourage the patient to participate in identifying and assessing his problem is to engage him as an active partner. . . . The power for accomplishing the tasks at hand, in ways that develop or expand personality, reside in the consent and understanding that motivate all persons concerned.
>
> (Peplau, 1952: p.23)

Therefore, advice, reassurance, suggestion, and persuasion are of little value in this assessment. Rather, my responses to my client should be undemanding and orientated towards his expression of feelings and views in order for him to become aware of them.

The assessment phase of Peplau's nursing process, along with the other phases are indicated in Fig. 4.3:

Orientation encounters 1–9
Identification encounters 7–16
Exploitation encounters 8–17
Resolution encounters 12–17

According to Peplau (1952), the assessment overlaps with the next phase, where

> the patient experiences degrees of the same feelings that operated at any earlier stage in his life. There is the complicating factor of chronological age and the imposition of cultural factors on the patient's view of himself. It may not be a simple achievement for the patient to permit expression of babylike feelings. It is as if the patient wishes to reassure himself that he has control beyond the extent indicated in his feelings.
>
> (Peplau, 1952: p.37)

This can be seen in the way, for example, Tom used my presence in family meetings to assert himself as he said he could not have done in the past (Fig. 4.3, encounter 6). Peplau (1985) believes that, other than the use of mechanical and chemical restraints, the only control a nurse has in relation to a client is the nurse's stimuli, i.e. language the nurse uses with the client. This stimulation, to which clients eventually respond, enables their self-correction of first their language and then thought.

Tom and I decided to look at the language we used with each other – first during assessment, then midway through the eight months of care, and at the end. We did this in two ways. Bits of sessions and sometimes whole sessions, including those with the family, were tape-recorded and later we would listen and discuss our impressions of ourselves. The second method was to tape-record Tom's descriptions of two unambiguous colour pictures. The transcripts were studied when they had been typed. This second method enabled us to look at his perceptions and anxiety, which arose in the process of his descriptions of what was going on in these two pictures. In our initial evaluation of this assessment method, Tom commented on how many of his sentences ended with questions. It appears clear in the repetitive questioning how anxious he is when asked to take the risk of answering a question which might be criticised –

we could hear and see the anxiety. The process of examining his perception in this way enabled me to better examine mine. I think Tom realised the extent of his being dominated by his mother because of his anxiety over doing wrong. This anxiety was reproduced in his responses to four questions asking him to describe the two pictures. (While the transcripts and pictures are not contained in this chapter, more will be said about this later.)

The assessment process appears to have enabled Tom, his mother, brother and sister, the social worker and myself, to actually see that Tom's mother had used what she considered her son's sickness to neglect her own development: she continued to mother, at age 70, as if she and her son were much younger. Tom, in increasing his expressiveness within the family, demonstrated an awareness of the control and influence in close relationships. Little is known about the personal adjustments that an individual might make in the process of becoming mentally ill – particularly with respect to people with whom they are intimate. But the interpersonal adjustments which occur are probably different from the adjustments made by the person who is seen to be sick. Tom used increased insight and anxiety to make changes in the way he managed himself with his mother, when I was present and when I was not (Fig. 4.3). During the assessment it became clear that, in the past, 'madness' (e.g., face-making and dancing around) was Tom's only resource that was effective in 'getting back' at his mother. During the client–nurse meetings, Tom recognised that pulling strange faces at home and jumping around in the kitchen were more tactics for dealing with his anger at his mother than ways of gaining satisfaction, such as going for walks or eating with his family.

The nursing assessment describes an in-appropriate use of a mothering role and the use by Tom's mother of highly-expressed emotion. If the assessment had missed these issues, it would be difficult to imagine that any helping strategies could get to grips with the disruptive conflicts between the needs of client, family, and carers on the one hand and the role demands of the social system on the other hand.

Tom used our relationship to facilitate forward movement of his personality in ways that replaced feelings of helplessness and powerlessness with feelings of creativeness, spontaneity, and productivity.

Analysis of strengths and weaknesses of the nursing offered
Strengths

An example of forward movement occurred when Tom decided to announce he wanted to leave home for the first time. This, combined with other signposts marking the end of the identification phase and beginning of exploitation, supports the value of Peplau's argument that the nurse should not impose theoretical, professional or personal values or standards on the client. The nurse learns how best to proceed, thereby freeing the client to recognise his identity, grow and develop his personality. Other examples supporting the strength of Peplau's model arise over the use of Tom's abusive language towards his mother. I referred Tom to his own perceptions of what was going on, asking that he express to me what he meant when swearing at his mother, rather than passing judgement on his intentions. As Peplau (1952) suggests,

> Exploiting what a situation offers gives rise to new differentiations of the problem and to the development and improvement of skills in interpersonal relations. New goals to be achieved through personal efforts can be projected.
>
> (Peplau, 1952: p.41)

The strength of the nurse–client relationship is perhaps best illustrated by the way in which we negotiated the Mental Illness Placements Panel questionnaire and subsequent interview, for the adult boarding-out scheme. Tom succeeded in obtaining a new place to live. It was evident as we both made new relationships among the Community Mental Health Team that he was freeing himself from identification with me and generating the strength and ability to stand upon his own feet.

These outcomes can be achieved only when all of the earlier phases are met in terms of psychological mothering: unconditional acceptance in a sustaining relationship that provides for full need-satisfaction ... shifting of power from the nurse to the patient as he becomes willing to delay gratification of his wishes and to expend his own efforts in achieving new goals.

(Peplau, 1952: p.40)

Resolution is a freeing process. Nursing helped to organise Tom's actions for more productive social activities and relationships of his own choosing. This stands in contrast to his early nursing care with me, which showed his achievement of satisfaction by smoking, eating, walking and sleeping. The nurse changes roles during the process of the care, from stranger, to resource person, to teacher, to surrogate, to counsellor (Peplau, 1952). The obvious support by Tom's brother and sister, and by his mother, lends credence to the use of this model of nursing.

This model supports my commitment and ability to use my knowledge base and enhance practical skills and formulate a specific direction for my nursing and teaching in mental health care.

Weaknesses of the nursing offered

There is an argument that by concentrating upon process Peplau neglects structure.

The split between task activities and human relationships skills is reflected in training and practice, and the reasons for this must be related in some sense to the overall structure of the hospital or to an even wider social context. Peplau, consistent with humanistic psychology in general, is weak in relating process to structure.

(Heyman and Shaw, 1984: p.34)

This criticism is perhaps most valid in the area of communication problems. These are seen not just in terms of skilled professional practice, but from conflicts and contradictions in the wider social structure in which nursing occurs. Heyman and Shaw argue that Peplau's perspective does not allow the individual nurse scope for changing the system in which she operates.

Similarly, Belcher and Fish (1985) suggest that today's nursing process views the recipient(s) of care collectively as a group, family, or community. Therefore, Peplau's model for nursing does not take into account the total environment.

Fawcett's (1984) review of theoretical frameworks does not even recognise interpersonal models. But, like Heyman and Shaw, she refers to 'characteristics of interaction models'. In the case of the Roy Adaptation model, Fawcett says this means the person is viewed as having a social component, referring to Roy's (1980) view that perception and the individual's behaviour relate to that of others on a group level. King's (1981) 'open systems model' is held by Fawcett to be characteristic of an interaction model. By this line of thinking, King relates perception to the 'social act of human interaction which occurs in the relationship between nurse and patient'.

Peplau avoids describing nursing in terms of a set of functions or tasks. Yet, she presents prescriptive statements about the potential of nursing (Belcher and Fish, 1985). She defines nursing as

a significant, therapeutic, interpersonal process ... an educative instrument, a maturing force, that aims to promote forward movement of personality in the direction of creative, constructive, productive, personal, and community living.

(Peplau, 1952: p.16)

Weakness in the Peplau model of nursing is associated with its emphasis upon the potential for personal growth by the client and the nurse. Consequently, the outcome of using such a model may depend upon the client's motivation, arguably the most problematic issue in psychiatric nursing *vis-à-vis* the nurse's role.

Peplau (1968) stipulates that the nurse should concentrate on the language items – the words – with which the patient does his thinking. She also expects an application of her model to include an examination of the patient's use of first person pronouns – I, me, mine – and 'global' pronouns used without naming their referents – we, they, us. Therefore, the tape-recordings of the story descriptions, which are not themselves included in this chapter, included an analysis of Tom's use of personal pronouns as a feature of his overall increase in the use of words to express his perceptions. However, the number of times he used personal pronouns shows no compatibility with the qualitative gains Tom made. He developed strategies for coping with his mother's highly-expressed emotion; he began to separate from her after 46 years; he began to manage productive relationships with 'new' people. He made these qualitative gains without significantly increasing his use of personal pronouns, while substantially increasing the amount of words he used overall.

Menuck and Seeman (1985) debunk Peplau's view on language altogether, saying a core problem has been the conceptual entangling of thought and language. The assumption that thought is reflected in language is not totally valid. It is not valid, they say, because people may have unspoken thoughts or say one thing and think another.

Concluding review of the use of Peplau's model

Sullivan's (1953) interpersonal theory of psychiatry was adapted for nursing by Peplau. Like Altschul's (1972) study, interpersonal relationships are identified as the source of therapeutic communication in psychiatric nursing. Bunch (1985), who did not use Peplau's nursing framework, said the main problem in implementing her concept of nursing was, as Altschul and he both found, that nurses are influenced to direct much of their attention to institutional business. That is, medicating people and 'talking shop' received more attention than the therapeutic engagement between nurse and client. Indeed, in the assessment of this case study with Tom, it would appear that the family dynamics were overlooked for a number of years. This raises a question of whether mental health nurses, in their professionalism, have limited potentials to understand or perceive how their actions are influenced by the social system or professional roles around them. It would seem that such constraints (against 'asking the family' and listening, for example) have to do with the business of the professional role, i.e. the medicating, the focus on attendance at the

mental health centre, and so on. Such a blunting effect upon a nurse's interface with a client may lend credence to the current fashion to deprofessionalise the mental health services, to 'normalise' the care of a client. To conclude this negative train of thought, the only prospect that Tom's therapeutic gains will have continuity may be in writing about our experience. The significant outcomes for Tom can hardly be ignored as an expression of the quality of the process. Furthermore, the learning value for me was outstanding.

Peplau did not want the nurse to interpret dynamics so much as to learn from the client the therapeutic impact of the nursing, for example the nurse's anxiety, or sense of guilt, might have an effect on the client which could impede or threaten growth. This awareness is essential in light of the real institutional and professional constraints of, traditionally, task-centred care and custodial roles. Also, the working out of the nurse's anxiety could prove too burdensome for the little-supervised nurse with many clients. I found a need for specific practical and theoretical mechanisms for dealing with intrapersonal issues in the interpersonal relationships. For me it was as if Peplau (1952, 1960) seemed to be using the learning aspects of her nursing model to avoid confronting the problem of perceptions being interpretations. By containing the nurse's role in this way, she could be seen to be neglecting nursing's therapeutic potential. To over-simplify the effect, it is as though the less the nurse intervenes, but uses Peplau's principles, the more effective is the client's self-development. The nurse as a person can feel she is being repressed in the aid of learning, as may be indicated in my decision to tell Tom's mother I could not tolerate her attack upon me.

It was apparent to me that internal communication was common right through the eight months. What distinguished this care from care in the past was the disciplined manner in which a shared meaning between nurse and client was pursued. By common, I mean, for instance, the way Tom 'read' my thoughts, beyond my verbal language (items) and before I had finished using words, i.e. responding by saying 'I think so' when I did not think he knew for sure. I would check this out by going back and referring to the issue again. He knew, because of non-verbal interpersonal aspects of our relationship, what I intended. He acted in unison with the intention, trusting in this rather than the apparent meaning of the language alone. Apart from our cultural, socio-economic and vocational differences, we were not operating on a language level but on an intuitive-dynamic level, as a product of our relationship, which could not be explained or supported by the Peplau construct alone. Furthermore, language *per se* may be a biased symbol on which to base a judgement about the meaning of what is being conveyed. Thus, the model of nursing will require a structure allowing interactive and dynamic understandings, which derive from within the individual nurse. You may, in mental illness, take the attitude that the intention of a person can differ from his action – the former having a social plausibility about it and the latter containing instinctual and uncontrollable features. Language may be based upon either intention or action or both; the point is that the study with Tom raises questions about the credibility of language *vis-à-vis* the shared meaning between nurse and client.

In its present state, the Peplau model for nursing has been used as an operating framework for introducing the ENB (1982) RMN syllabus in some areas, and in post-registration courses for mental health care nursing. Therefore, we can expect to see further evaluations of this model on a wider scale and in different settings and situations. The implications of my work with Tom suggest that such an evaluation should be rigorous and the Peplau model divested of its weaknesses and developed on its strengths. Secondly, the transition from mental hospitals to community-based care finds the nurse and client having to re-identify their role and priorities in care. Peplau's model poses a strong identity for nurses who are engaged in the changes of developing new mental health services. There is a growing commitment for a partnership with users of services and potential users in future services (IAMHW, 1985).

Tom said he most enjoyed learning to count money. He is proud of his decision to move out and be independent of his mother. He sees her frequently. He also indicated that he can continue to use a relationship to a satisfactory end, as far as he is concerned. He has made forward movement in the four psychological tasks in the nursing model: learning to count on others without longing for dependency, delaying instant satisfaction for higher satisfaction, identifying himself and developing skills in participation.

Fig. 4.3   Care plan. Sample extracts of meetings during an eight month period, using a nursing process format for recording/evaluating interpersonal relationships (Peplau, 1950: p.308)

Responses of the client (Location)	Responses of the nurse	Analysis and speculations of the nurse two days later
1 *Mental Health Centre*		
	Two weeks ago, when we met with your social worker, mother and brother, people seemed to be talking about you more than we were comfortable with – remember our talking about this?	The nurse seemed to have a certain direction in mind rather than focusing specifically on the client's 'language items' (and values) as Peplau (1952) suggested. Her technique (1960) needed more concentration here by the nurse. However, this was a shared orientation during assessment in the nursing psycho-therapeutic process. By the end, the client stated his perceptions, which were only a hypothesis in the nurse's mind (based primarily on the first family meeting at their home).
TOM: Yeah, ah, I think that's right.	Does this occur a lot, and what does it make you feel like?	
It does, and I feel ashamed.	You said last week when we met with the social worker that you wanted me to help you to speak your own mind and stand on your own feet . . .	
Yeah, that's right . . .	What are your thoughts about doing that when people, by your own admission, are running you down (to use your phrase)?	
It's like here, at the Centre, I often feel bored or that I want to run off . . .	What do you actually do?	
Here, ya mean?	Yeah, okay, here.	
Maybe have a smoke with Frank (a friend), or a coffee, or go out for a walk, but it's not like my mum – she really gets on my nerves; I can't do nothin' right.		
2 *Mental Health Centre*		
	The nurses had told me your name was Sid and the social workers said it was Tom.	The nurse's first impression of Tom, at 46, was of a person behaving like an adolescent, insofar as the adolescent crisis is about *finding* an adult integrity of the self, whereas the midlife crisis is highlighted by a sense of loss – of old enjoyable capacities and loss of capacity to procreate (Rayner, 1978). Therefore, the nurse's orientation to the client would be based not so much on what Rayner called a 'normal depressive crisis' but on a 'normal schizoid' one.
TOM: I decided to be called Tom; it just came to me. I never asked anyone to call me Sid and have never used my first name, Cyril. I was once called Ray, my middle name, but I didn't like it.		
3 *Mental Health Centre*		
	I don't like it when you blow smoke in my face, although I don't mind if you smoke occasionally. You were smoking hard and sweating during the first part of our first meeting, remember?	However, the orientation and assessment continues to inform the nurse's objectivity through the client's subjective viewpoints. Regarding 'You do what you think' – Peplau (1952) insisted on the nurse being nondirective in a nonjudgemental way. The nurse's
TOM: Yeah . . . I'll put it out if you like.	You do what you think. You smoke when you're uncomfortable?	

Fig. 4.3 (continued)

Responses of the client (Location)	Responses of the nurse	Analysis and speculations of the nurse two days later
I guess so.	Well, why do you like going for walks?	attempt to identify with the client's experience was intended to strengthen a relationship between the two, which would act as a catalyst for change if and when the client wished to act for change. Nurturing a relationship in this way would promote Peplau's (1952) identification phase of the nursing process, during which planning would become more apparent.
It makes me happy.	Is that why you dance around at home and also sometimes make faces.	
Yes.	Even though it annoys mum?	
I 'spose it does.	These things that give you satisfaction seem very important to you.	
I need to do these things that make me happy.	I need that too.	
I get happy with my record player. I get happy when I go out sometimes. Frank and a couple of other friends here make me happy. But my mum doesn't make me happy.		

4 Mental Health Centre

	What can I help you with?	The nurse focused on the client's language items, inducing assessment generated by the client. However, a current question in the nurse's mind, having accepted and agreed nursing with Tom, was this: who was the 'patient' really? From the paucity of client-centred information in nursing and medical notes, it seemed that what this nurse had experienced with the family had not been taken into account (although initial medical diagnosis of schizophrenia predated conclusive research into effects of high expressed emotion in families: Brown *et al.*, 1958, 1962, 1972; Vaughn and Leff, 1976; Vaughn *et al.*, 1982). Nevertheless, familiarity with existing psychiatric nursing, psychological, and sociological research would have made an educated guess and straightforward literary enquiry a matter of urgent professional responsibility as part of assessment. Mother was a significant influence in Tom's lost control – both of himself and his social relations. His sweating early in the sessions was related to issues 'hotting up' internally, so that cooling down successfully with the nurse was meant to be a practical strategy using a relationship therapeutically.
TOM: Everything!	I can't be a mother to you.	
I wish you'd be my father!	Father?	
I like him better; she's a bit awkward.	A 'bit'?	
Well, ah, I hit 'er on the way to Mrs Webbs' . . .	Bonfire night.	
Yeah, Saturday; well, ah, I picked up a tobacco box from the floor of the bus and took a butt outta it; mum grabbed it away and threw it on the floor and stomped on it . . . then I hit 'er on the shoulder . . .	Could you have used words instead?	
Yes, I think so.	Which ones?	
I dunno.	What did you feel like before you hit her and after?	
Uh, angry, but it makes me feel bad after.	Could you say 'I am angry . . .'?	
I am angry . . .	To mum, I mean.	
I dunno.	You remember when we first talked a month ago, you said it would be 'impossible' (to use your word) to say what you felt inside yourself for fear of it leading to further dispute. Well, if you said what was going on inside yourself, do you think it	

Fig. 4.3   (continued)

Responses of the client (Location)	Responses of the nurse	Analysis and speculations of the nurse two days later
	would 'stop the fire' (as we called it) getting too hot and impossible to control?	The nurse has a sense here of compromising a focus on the client's language items to clarify the assessment – whether the nurse and client share a perception of what the client wants to 'work on'. The first tape-recorded description of the two colour pictures (for evaluating the assessment) was two weeks ago. This has helped to demonstrate when and where the client is too anxious to think and therefore allows the nurse's interventions to be more effective. The tapes are replayed after recording by the client and nurse, and when the transcribing is finished by the nurse, the two people study them visually, with a shared view of the perceptual clarity and cognitive understanding of the client discussed with the nurse.
I think it'd be possible to use words; sometimes it makes me sad the way mum nags me, but I've not been able to tell her.	Why do you think these arguments arise over food and tobacco and your walks? Do you recall saying these are things which give you satisfaction?	
Yeah, I like me food 'n fags . . .	What do you do when you don't attend the Centre here?	
Walkin' . . . the park, maybe, or if I'm home, ta shops, but mum says I can't carry money or somebody will take it off me.	Can I be of any help to her; is she hurt? Did you make her a hot water bottle last night, as usual?	
Yeah, and she said prayers for me and I gave her a kiss.		

5 *Mental Health Centre*		
	I notice you didn't come in smoking today, and once more you haven't smoked during this hour.	The nurse had tried to make a health-statement in previous sessions and also establish the nurse's identity and now wondered whether the client's action was a result of the former, just to please the nurse, or the client's stated reason, which the nurse accepted.
TOM: I guess I just didn't feel like it; we been talkin' so much I just didn't think to.	Yes, I enjoyed hearing about Flo' – reminded me of Pooch, my dog when I was little.	

6 *Mental Health Centre*		
	You seem quite heated up today, is something the matter?	This meeting seemed intimate and more shared than previous sessions. Tom used the time to offer problems and used the nurse to consider possible strategies for prospective solutions – an indication that the identification phase of the nursing process was well underway and plans being made in the relationship for a course that the nursing would support. More 'response' from the client and use by the nurse of items he 'brought' – demonstrating in Peplau's (1952) terms the use in relationships of language items as they provide a verbal base for the development of stimulation and motivation for the client who uses his anxiety as part of growth and development of personality, with the help and guidance of a nurse.
TOM: Rachel was outta control and smashed a cup against the wall and I thought she was gonna break a window . . .	Your brother's daughter; you and mum stayed at their house over the weekend then?	
Yeah, and Rachel went mad; my brother got a letter and he just read it and Rachel kept going on at him and he had been going on at 'er 'bout this letter or summit.	What did you do?	
Nothin'.	What did you think of Rachel? What did you want to say to her?	
To stop it, to stop it; she was a bas . . .	Go on . . .	
She was a bastard, a real bastard.	Does your brother get on to her like mum gets on to you?	

Fig. 4.3 (continued)

Responses of the client (Location)	Responses of the nurse	Analysis and speculations of the nurse two days later
Yes. Mum calls me a silly bastard 'n all. Last week I called her a silly cow but I can't think why.	And you, what names do you call her? Why wouldn't you tell your brother by using words how worried you are that, as you've said before, he stays away from work because of his problems with Rachel?	Tom was dressed slovenly – he had a blue pullover for the third Monday evening in succession, with two lighter shirts beneath, one hanging below his outer pullover and over his trousers. The trousers looked as though they were stained at the knee. He said that's where he rubs his hands on his trousers.
I would do, I would do, but I'm worried he'll get back at me. Yeah, well I do want to learn.	I notice you're using more words with people in my presence. Is this deliberate, are you doing this on purpose?	

7 *Mental Health Centre*

	You mentioned before that mum gives you money of a day and some cigarettes each morning. What do you think about this system? Could you manage more of your £30-odd a week? For example on clothes? When we first met you were all dressed up, but for the past several weeks you've worn almost the same clothes.	Tom's statements of what goes on in his life identifies to him and verifies to the nurse that perceptions are understood and particularly that the nurse's observations are tested against the client's perceptions. *The client appears from time to time not to want to focus on issues which the nurse sees as pertinent, but the nurse is influenced by Peplau's (1952) underlying interest in anxiety arising from interferences with the motivation to be satisfied. The nurse and client had spoken of alternative goals for satisfaction – conversation rather than excessive smoking, for instance. Having said this, and notwithstanding constraints of time, the nurse should dwell on the client's offering until the client is prepared to develop his thinking.
TOM: I asked me mum to buy me another pair of shoes but she never. But she said I could keep me Christmas bonus.	Tom, can you count money?	
No, not much – I usually get the wrong change when she sends me to the store and then I have to go back again.	What do you think?	
Well, I suppose I should learn if you could help me.	I can help and perhaps we can talk to the workers here – to see if money as a subject might fit into one of the groups, eh?	The nurse was aware in this session of using language items Tom brought, rather than working on thought or behaviour disorder the nurse might have assumed.
Yeah, that's a good idea. I'm smokin' roll-ups now; look. But I haven't smoked any yet with you.*	There is the problem you mentioned of wanting to run away when it comes to attending groups here.	The nurse continues to shape issues as part of the identification phase of the nursing process.
I just come and drink and smoke, yeah. I'll try to go to the groups. I do want to go. I used to go, but I guess I just got bored with it.	Have you ever told anyone that?	
No.	Why not?	
I dunno.	Is it the same reason you don't tell your brother you're worried about him – is it just too risky?	

Fig. 4.3   (continued)

Responses of the client (Location)	Responses of the nurse	Analysis and speculations of the nurse two days later
I'm afraid of what it might lead to – I just don't know what would happen.	It is helping you decide to discuss things like this.	
Yeah, it is, I think it is, yeah.		

8   *Client's home*

MUM: Stop fussing over the tea, Tom. Come here and put the cups out (as if speaking to the social worker and nurse): the one thing he can do well is make a cup of tea. But he fusses too much with the cups, watch.

TOM: I want to have a cigarette (reaching through mum's grip on his arm, retrieving a cigarette despite her restraint).

MUM: Those two don't smoke, ask them if they mind you smoking . . . they wouldn't say, *they're* visitors.

TOM: Well, I'll move over here (out of the way) and sit down and light up.

MUM: He shouldn't smoke really, you know, it's bad for your health.

Maybe there are other reasons why you smoke Tom.

Tom behaves as though he is a receptive container (Peplau, 1952) for mother's anguish. Despite the denigration and harranguing the nurse believes that Tom is already beginning to *exploit* his therapeutic relationship by showing he is willing and prepared with his nurse present to verbally assert himself. This client action indicates the third phase of Peplau's (1952) nursing process. Although a passive recipient of these apparent exaggerations for the moment, Tom seemed to be waiting for his chance to act, because, based on his descriptions of past incidents with mother, if the nurse was not present he would probably be storming back at her or else 'winding her up' with his dancing or face-making which ignored her demandingness.* It was interesting to note at this point that mother just sat contented when the nurse looked across at her with a 'questionmark-face'.

MUM: He does all sorts here, ya know . . . dancing around, with them old people downstairs – what if the floor fell in – and making faces in that mirror . . . he don't do a thing around here.

TOM: It makes me happy dancing and making faces . . . I do some things here, you just don't like 'em.

MUM: Tom can't even wash out a milk bottle properly, never mind take them tablets of his on time.

Who's responsible for the medication?

TOM: Well, she is.

Who's responsible for the money in this household?*

TOM: Well, she is.

Is there anything mum is not responsible for?

TOM: No, she's responsible for everything.

Are you both saying the other should be more sharing in responsibility and caring for what makes the other happy?

Fig. 4.3   (continued)

Responses of the client (Location)	Responses of the nurse	Analysis and speculations of the nurse two days later
BOTH: Yes. Yes, that's right.	Would mum be willing to share responsibility more with Tom?	
MUM: Like what?		
SOCIAL WORKER: Like, for example, the cooking. Could you, even if the washing up wasn't quite to your exact routine and standard, could you give Tom the opportunity of doing it, without this back-biting.		

9   *Client's home*

BROTHER: Tom has tried to empty the rubbish for mum this week but mum wouldn't have it.		The nurse's main task this session was to listen – observation precedes the interpretation of collected data (Peplau, 1952). The nurse decided to maintain a 'low profile' to allow the family to interact as much as possible, letting them know, however, that Tom was supported but trying not to take sides while allowing a strategy for resolution to evolve based on values which the family as client would express.
MUM: Well, he don't take it down when he should. He shoulda taken it down the other night after he had fish and chips here, but he didn't so I took it down. We live with other people in this building and well it smells doesn't it.		
BROTHER: Mum you've got to let him do this for himself; you're the problem, not 'im!		The nurse was beginning to feel the strain of having no supervision in which to discuss the nurse's responses in light
MUM: It's not just that, his memory is bad; he don't remember things, that's the real problem, his memory is bad. He forgets to check his change at the store and gets money short.	Tom, can you count money?	of the psychological problems within the family, especially involving mother and client. The nurse's 'clinical supervisor' for the third year of the Diploma of Nursing was absent, on extended sick leave. However, brief discussions with a fellow diploma student about some of the issues and with friends who were graduates from the Institute of Group Analysis, would prove helpful without impinging on the confidentiality of the work.
TOM: No, I don't know how to count very well, specially backwards when you get coppers 'n things like given you back.		
MUM: Well that's just it, ya see, I keep telling him to go to the Centre ta learn things and all he does he goes there with the likes a Frank, who takes things off him, cigarettes and money. Explain this, why does he come to me and ask me about you, 'Is he comin' today mum, is he?' when he knows damn well you are, huh?	I'm here to help you with what you've asked of me and with what we've agreed, not to referee fights or use me to abuse each other – but to help you develop ways of being together which you both find satisfactory. Tom in particular asked for support in telling you, which he has done on several occasions now, that he is unhappy and dissatisfied with your criticism of him. He has also said he wants to help care for you if you will allow it.	
TOM: That's right.		

Fig. 4.3   (continued)

Responses of the client (Location)	Responses of the nurse	Analysis and speculations of the nurse two days later
BROTHER: This means one person having a job to do and seeing it through to its goal and the other person accepting, like leaving Tom to do the rubbish and hoovering and meals he's agreed to.		

10   *Client's home*

Responses of the client (Location)	Responses of the nurse	Analysis and speculations of the nurse two days later
MUM: Tom was a *good boy* during this week.	What do you mean?	During this session Tom is passively containing gross exaggerations, but now beginning to throw them out, exploiting the nursing resource again. The nurse is reminded of two main developmental issues which may feature in the anxious way mother projects her feelings:
MUM: He broke everything he touched. He dropped everything he picked up.		
TOM: Yeah, I didn't seem to be able to hang on to anything.		(1) The extent to which she blames Tom for her son's death in a London air raid during World War II – the boys had been playing whilst walking to the shops with mother. When Tom and mother mentioned this incident, during the orientation/assessment stage of the nursing process, they did not indicate any 'surface' or thought-about blame and below-the-surface or unconscious feelings did not seem to the nurse appropriately accessible. However, there were possible non-verbal indications that mother resented Tom for his little brother bolting off across the street, where he died in the blast. Mother was buried in rubble, she said, on 'her' side of the street, leaving Tom unscathed in the middle.
MUM: He broke the clock I got when we were married.		
TOM: Oh, it wasn't that old, was it?		
MUM: Well, maybe not, that one, but it was old.	Is that what you mean by 'everything', to use your word, one treasured clock?	
MUM: Oh, that's not all – he raised his fist to me the other night 'n all.		
TOM: I was listening to the radio and she kept going on at me that it was too loud . . .		
MUM: . . . It was too loud for the Jones' downstairs and also he was singing over the radio and I couldn't hear the story about caffeine.	So you had a verbal fight and then the old clock broke . . . has it helped taking half an hour to tell somebody else what happened?	(2) The second main developmental issue the nurse is reminded of by mother's apparently distorted indictments is old age. She is presented with threats to her well-being from two directions:
TOM: Um, it's not as bad as it sounds.		(i) firstly, from the deterioration of bodily functions (widespread 'small deaths' caused by shrinkage of bodily functions: cell tissue is not replaced as in youth, so that hair thins, skin and muscles lose their vibrance, blood circulation malfunctions and brain cells die);
MUM: It's not fighting.		

11   *Client's home*

Responses of the client (Location)	Responses of the nurse	Analysis and speculations of the nurse two days later
	Those gestures you're making with your mouth, are they rude words Tom made during the week?	
MUM: I can't say them . . . but he knows!	I'm not surprised you're dealing with issues between yourselves, nor that it's unpleasant getting them resolved; how can I help?	(ii) secondly, from social expectations that she will become useless on account of her age, irrespective of her real capacities. Mother has clearly indicated to the nurse that 'Well, if I can't be helpful in this way, then I may as well
MUM: He called me a fucking cunt.		

Fig. 4.3 (continued)

Responses of the client (Location)	Responses of the nurse	Analysis and speculations of the nurse two days later
TOM: I didn't mean it, it just come out.		pack it in now', i.e. her mothering role is a way she does not have to accept the shrinkage of her life, although her depressive feelings with ageing are masked by the anger she projects. Beneath this overlay, there may be some denied issues to do with her husband's death. Although this occurred a number of years ago, her grief or lack of grief may become evident to her as part of the outcome of Tom's nursing and the surface issue of her ageing. Her husband was an invalid for some time before he died.
MUM: He wanted two packs of cigarettes, not just one.		
TOM: Well, me brother has two packs a day.		
MUM: It was Wednesday, after he collected his money. When I said no, he pulled a ten-pound note out of my hand and called me that, and also he threw a tea bag at me.		
TOM: I never hit you with it, I threw it at the door behind.		
MUM: Did you see that show on telly the other night . . . what was it sciphre . . . well, 'at's the way they get when they're psyckiatric. Well, I can put him in a home if I want to, you know. Now I ask you, at my age should I have to put up with this; what can I do?	Once again, the argument seems to be over something which Tom gets satisfaction from. While I agree that smoking isn't healthy, we have seen that what makes Tom happy you are not satisfied with – and in the case of smoking you are a pack-a-day smoker who probably has some understanding of the habit. Let me draw a picture to illustrate my advice . . . you can see that when these goals to satisfaction are interfered with, then there arises frustration, conflict, anxiety, and possibly in the long run a complete lack of control and physical fighting.	Mother's exaggerated criticism is the pretence of avoiding dependency, to some extent, in old age, while at the same time reinforcing Tom's longing for dependency (Peplau, 1952), which the nursing intervention is correcting.

As ego-functioning and the sense of self tend to shrink, one would expect primitive, less integrated patterns of thought and feeling to emerge. This regression is manifest not only in mother's generalised fearfulness (expressed in Tom's going for walks), but also in her tendencies to use projective mechanisms (Rayner, 1978). |
SISTER: Yes, I remember my brother saying that during the session he was in that you had talked about this and agreed that Tom and Mum would be individually responsible for everyday jobs and try not to be so critical of each other's work.	Do you two remember that also?	
BOTH: Yeah, uh huh.		
SISTER: Tom is a smashing bloke on his own, but when he's with you Mum he's a different person – there's nothin' but argument.		
MUM: What! This is not all my fault you know.		
SISTER: I know this hurts you Mum, but you know I've said it before.		

Fig. 4.3   (continued)

Responses of the client (Location)	Responses of the nurse	Analysis and speculations of the nurse two days later
MUM: He wouldn't even kiss me the other night. He said 'Why should *I* kiss *you*.'	Is the idea about getting satisfaction through achieving goals without a lot of interference . . . is this idea making sense to you?	
TOM: Don't go to sleep Mum . . .		
MUM: . . . Rubbish, I'm listening; it's like what we was talkin' about you doing the rubbish when you seen fit and me tryin' not to complain about the fish smell.		

12   *Client's home*

MUM: Tom's not kissing me goodnight at all and he's called me that word again, twice on Thursday night, once in the kitchen and from the bottom of the stairs. He almost hurt me when he slammed the kitchen door on the way out, and if he is like this a neighbour or I might call the police – if I'm hurt. This is how he was those years ago when he went to the hospital.	I understand your alarm and suggest Tom and I meet now at the Centre for a while. He is having trouble attending groups there and also this would take the pressure off you both – I expect that while you both may get emotional relief from the feelings and attitudes you express, it's a painful process, but it has informed our working together.	The nurse saw a potentially untherapeutic pattern emerging if the short series of family meetings were to continue at present and also wished to indicate to the individuals their responsibilities for stable relationships, by deciding to continue with the one client rather than by taking on the family as client, at the suggestion of Tom's brother.
MUM: I like you to come to the house; you can come any time you like. I don't want you to go away . . . thinking we have arguments all the time.	Oh, I'd like to be with you again, too, but Tom and I have some work to do, both on delaying satisfactions sometimes and on being in groups.	
TOM: I do want to learn; I went to the Centre on Thursday.	Did you go because your injection was due?	
TOM: Yeah, I had it . . . Really, I would much rather live on my own.		A further, and the most significant, exploitation of his nursing resource. Separation from mother will need to be explored individually. The nurse's position is that even when emotional factors might be considered at a minimum, talking about one's own problems, in an atmosphere calculated to make defensiveness unnecessary, tends to clarify the adjustments which one must make, to give a more clear-cut picture of problems and difficulties, to give possible choices their true values in terms of one's own feelings (Rogers, 1942).
MUM: He didn't come back on Thursday night and I worried to death not knowing where he was walking the streets or laying dead . . .		
TOM: I stayed at my brother's.	Had you thought about leaving home before?	
TOM: For years, but I never said nothing.	Have you two ever talked about it?	
TOM: No, my brother said he might be able to find me a place sometime – that was years ago – I would like to move.		

Fig. 4.3 (continued)

Responses of the client (Location)	Responses of the nurse	Analysis and speculations of the nurse two days later
13 *Client's home*		
MUM: Well, if he leaves, he'll never come back . . .		Following feedback on our meeting with the Mental Illness Housing Panel and their favourable inclination for Tom to be offered Adult Boarding Out accommodation, the reality of his leaving is impacting on mother. Clearly, the stigma she associates with the label of mental illness has been a disadvantage if not a handicap to possible opportunities of independent decision-making in the past – hence, for example, his fury after brief support and insight, after it was clear that another person would think well of him. The sick role has also reinforced the mothering role to the detriment of her own development as it's got tangled emotionally with issues of ageing. The nursing plan has been implemented through Tom's decision to be assertive, independent-minded and expressive, culminating in his use of the nurse to coordinate a complex of other care workers in executing the social services machinery necessary to gain a housing place.
TOM: Oh, I would . . .		
MUM: No he wouldn't, and I wouldn't want him back either. He should stay with me until I die then go into a psyckiatric hospital, because that's what he is – sciphrenia.	The Community Mental Health Team will probably support Tom's application for a shared house. Have you mentioned this Tom?	
TOM: Yes; I would come and visit you in the week.	I have said before that Tom does not view himself as a sick or diseased person, either mentally or physically. I do not view Tom as sick either, nor does the doctor who he sees four times a year.	

14 *Mental Health Centre*		
TOM: Mum wants to know how much the rent will be at my new house. My brothers and sister also asked. Mum said would you write it down on a piece of paper. I said it was £49 as far as I can remember.	I can't remember either; I think it depends on the kind of accommodation – you'll have to ask that new social worker next time we meet. Didn't she say we'd be seeing a place this month?
Yeah, that's right; it's just that they wanted it written down.	I think you could tell them not to worry because, as I remember it, you would be paid more to cater for the rent, isn't that so?
Yes. When am I going to move? Will it be a house, will it? When will it be?	Well, once again, what they seemed to be saying at the housing panel we went to is that it's up to you. I mean, whether you show them at the house that your practical and thinking and expressive skills are sufficient, for example handling money and managing with food.
You're helping me to learn to count money . . .	Yes, but you're not using the Centre to support our work; we had agreed you would attend at least two groups, for example. Do you

Fig. 4.3   (continued)

Responses of the client (Location)	Responses of the nurse	Analysis and speculations of the nurse two days later
	come here when we arrange to meet here only because you think I can, alone, help you?	
Well, I guess so.	I can't teach you what you need to know; I can help, but you need to learn from others. My advice is, if you want to demonstrate your competence, use the Centre, use other people.	
So, I need to work harder.	I would say it needs to come from within you – not from me. You have replaced some smoking in our meetings with gaining satisfaction from what we do together; you've used this with your mother; you've spoken your mind; you've decided to be independent. *You* have done these things.	

15   *Client's home*

	I can tell by your gesturing again while Tom is busy with the tea that you two have had some critical moments together.	
MUM: He was drinking straight out of a milk bottle, contaminating it; he threw a Bic razor blade at me . . .		
TOM: I didn't, I threw it against the door and it never hit you . . .		
MUM: He messed up a towel by wiping the mirror the way he did . . .		
TOM: You never told me to use the wiping-up cloth until after . . .		
MUM: He's been slamming the doors and I will call the police if it doesn't stop; he was singing louder and louder over the radio, and the other day he was short-changed even though I wrote out explicit instructions; on top of that he used indecent language. And his brother scolded him for breathing over his daughter's tea while he (Tom) was drinking and eating biscuits from his tea.	You are driving *me* up the wall, with your verbally and physically aggressive ways of expressing yourself. It has upset me and I can't concentrate. It's not that I have a bad memory or that I am sick. You have abused me and yourself in this way – yourself because I can tell from seeing your legs that you are not resting twice a day as I suggested; is this right?	The nurse decided it would be ingenuine to try and conceal the damage experienced by such acrimonious and threatening attack. Further, that concealment of feelings may damage the sense of trust the nurse had obviously developed with the family.
BOTH: Yeah.	Once more, you've asked my advice in the past on how to stop this	Slow, strong words from the nurse, as with Tom previously, having to show the

Fig. 4.3 (continued)

Responses of the client (Location)	Responses of the nurse	Analysis and speculations of the nurse two days later
	chronic painful quarrelling and unkindness towards yourselves and others and seem to have neglected that advice, although I understand how very hard it is for you to find new ways of coping. I suggested you need to look at what part you play, Mum, in these arguments. In my view you are both equally responsible. I can see and you have each said how you play on the other.	limits of the nurse's perceived responsibility and in so doing indicate their part, based on what they had put into the 'open' and verified with the nurse.
MUM: Tom is totally different with other people.	I know.	
MUM: I'm only trying to help.	We have looked at several examples in the past, about how you do this in a way which provokes anger and today is another example.	Again, mother defends behaviours which her siblings condemned in family meetings, behaviours which serve as a defensive mechanism to avoid dealing with herself and her ageing.
MUM: Yes, I am not too old to know what's happening.	Tom, have you mentioned to Mum that we are visiting local shops today to look at items for sale and their prices, as part of learning to count money?	
TOM: Yeah, I have. We better go now.	I wonder Tom whether your Mum is hard of hearing to the extent that one reason she may talk loudly and appear aggressive is because of the extent of her failing hearing? What do you think?	The pair were now out of the house, heading for the local shops. The client and nurse used part of their weekly Centre meetings to practice counting money, by using the nurse's 'piggy-bank' contents of coppers to establish the principle of counting and thinking in tens.
TOM: I don't think she's hard of hearing.		

16   *Mental Health Centre*

TOM: She wound me up by asking me if I wound up my clock, when she must have seen me wind it that morning.	And so you started this one?	Peplau (1952, 1968, 1978) predicts radical 'swings' in the process of the identification, and in the exploitation, of the nursing process, as pre-adolescent and adolescent behaviours emerge along
Yeah, I called her a c-u-n-t.	Was that all she did, ask you if you wound your clock.	with intermingling of needs and a shuttling back and forth, when rapid shifts in behaviour that express mixed
Yeah.	What did you feel like before calling Mum a c-u-n-t.	needs makes observation more complex. Peplau predicts that behaviour during the exploitation phase is more like that of
Wild.	What does that mean?	an adolescent – striking the balance is difficult, between a need to be
Well, angry. I just let it off, I guess.	And as usual you felt what?	dependent, as during illness, and a need to be independent, as following recovery.
Yes, sad, but also disappointed that after all our work with using words I didn't say angry instead of c-u-n-t.	Well, you're certainly learning. I've said some things to you and Mum that made me sad. Have I ever	Nursing has the task of understanding

Fig. 4.3   (continued)

Responses of the client (Location)	Responses of the nurse	Analysis and speculations of the nurse two days later
	made you feel wild so that you thought I was a c-u-n-t.	what gives rise to these shifts in behaviour.
Oh no, Bill, you don't make me feel like that! No. In fact, the next morning she said 'good morning' to me. By the way, she is resting on her bed now in the afternoons.	Do you think Mum is *responsible* for your anger.	The actual words Tom sometimes uses, especially when he's not consciously aware of his thinking, tend to contradict his actual feelings, at least to the extent this is based on the nurse's experience with him. Therefore, the nurse is attempting to use a language item such as c-u-n-t and relate it to the client's internal agenda (Peplau, 1952), so that the reality of his growing cognitive understanding is what gets externalised.

17   *En route to what will be the client's new home*

TOM: It's the Queen's Birthday today; you been watchin' it on the telly? Whadda do then come all the way over here on the train? You know me Mum's still at my brother's. That's right, I been on me own. Yeah. No 'cause I ain't seen her. Fine, I been buying from the shops 'n countin' me money back . . . an on the telly a whole lot of children sang for the Queen. No, I just been a little lonely, that's all. No, I haven't been for two weeks. Who's gonna be there tonight? Yeah, I had a shave last night; at first I didn't think it would come off! I think I'll be alright; I still wanna move. What's the number again? Yeah, that's it: 64 Grove Road.	No, I just moved to a new flat and nothin's working yet. What happened? Yeah, only had to change once, though. What do you mean, she never came back since Easter? That's a surprise; is she okay? Does she know you're going to see this house tonight? How've you been on your own? I bet that was a spectacle. Has being on your own given you any second thoughts about wanting to be there at Mum's house? Haven't you been to the Centre? The social worker, the landlady and landlord, and the five fellows living there? How do you feel? You look spruced up. Sixty-four.	This extract is from part of a conversation *en route* to the house placement interview. This talk drew attention to the client, seemingly because of his need to be heard and clear in his own mind, over the drone and noise of the surrounding crowd and town sounds. It reminded the nurse again of the complicating factors of chronological age and the imposition of cultural factors on the client's view of himself. It seemed until now a simple achievement for the client to permit expression of babylike feelings, as if he wished to reassure himself that he has control beyond the extent indicated in his feelings. His nurse should be perceptive of both – the psychological feelings and the cultural counter-feelings and attempts to help him experience both with a minimum of interference to the outcome of his nursing care.

References

Altschul AT 1972 *Patient–Nurse Interaction: A Study of Interaction Patterns in Acute Psychiatric Wards.* Churchill Livingstone, Edinburgh.

Altschul AT (Ed) 1985 *Psychiatric Nursing: Recent Advances in Nursing 12.* Churchill Livingstone, Edinburgh.

Baert AE 1980 Why do we need alternatives? *World Hospitals,* 16, 4: 19–20.

Barnes E (Ed) 1968 *Psychosocial Nursing: Studies from the Cassel Hospital.* Tavistock Publications, London.

Baruch G & Treacher A 1978 *Psychiatry Observed.* Routledge & Kegan Paul, London.

Belcher JR & Fish LJB 1985 Hildegard E Peplau. In *Nursing Theories: The Base for Professional Nursing Practice,* 2nd Ed, pp. 50–68. JB George (Ed). Prentice-Hall, Englewood Cliffs, New Jersey.

Beck CM, Rawlins RP & Williams SR (Eds) 1984 *Mental Health – Psychiatric Nursing: A Holistic Life-Cycle Approach.* CV Mosby Company, St Louis.

Brown GW, Carstairs GM & Topping GG 1958 Posthospital adjustment of chronic mental patients. *Lancet,* 2: 685–689.

Brown GW, Monck EM, Carstairs GM & Wing JK 1962 Influence of family life on the course of schizophrenic illness. *British Journal of Preventive and Social Medicine,* 16: 55–68.

Brown GW, Birley JLT & Wing JK 1972 Influence of family life on the course of schizophrenia. *British Journal of Psychiatry,* 121: 241–258.

Bunch EG 1985 Therapeutic communication: Is it possible for psychiatric nurses to engage in this on acute psychiatric wards? In *Psychiatric Nursing,* pp.43–62. AT Altschul (Ed). Churchill Livingstone, Edinburgh.

Burnard P 1986 Picking up the pieces. *Nursing Times,* 28, 17: 37–39.

Chenitz CW & Swanson JM 1985 Surfacing nursing process: A method for generating nursing theory from practice. *Journal of Advanced Nursing,* 9: 205–215.

Davis BD 1984 What is the nurse's perception of the patient?. In *Understanding Nurses: The Social Psychology of Nursing,* pp.67–80. S Skevington (Ed). John Wiley & Sons, Chichester.

English National Board 1982 *Syllabus of Training, Professional Register: Part 3 (Registered Mental Nurse).* English and Welsh National Boards for Nursing, Midwifery and Health Visiting.

Diers D 1979 *Research in Nursing Practice.* JP Lippincott, Philadelphia.

Fawcett J 1984 *Analysis and Evaluation of Conceptual Models of Nursing.* FA Davis, Philadelphia.

Fitzpatrick J, Whall A, Johnston R & Floyd I (Eds) 1982 *Nursing Models and their Psychiatric Mental Health Applications.* Robert J Brady Co, Bowie, Maryland.

Harré R, Clark D & DeCarlo N 1985 *Motives and Mechanisms: An Introduction to the Psychology of Action.* Methuen, London.

Heyman G & Shaw M 1984 Looking at relationships in nursing. In *Understanding Nurses: The Social Psychology of Nursing,* pp.29–46. S Skevington (Ed). John Wiley & Sons, Chichester.

Interdisciplinary Association of Mental Health Workers 1985 *Organisational Handbook.* IAMHW, University of Surrey.

Kelley HH, Berscheid E, Christensen A, Harvey JH, Huston TL, Levinger G, McClintock E, Peplau LA & Peterson DR 1983 *Close Relationships.* WH Foreman & Co, New York.

King IM 1981 *A Theory for Nursing: Systems, Concepts, Process.* John Wiley & Sons, New York.

Llewelyn SP 1984 The cost of giving: Emotional growth and emotional stress. In *Understanding Nurses: The Social Psychology of Nursing,* pp.49–65. S Skevington (Ed). John Wiley & Sons, Chichester.

McFarlane EA 1980 Nursing theory: The comparison of four theoretical proposals. *Journal of Advanced Nursing,* 5: 3–19.

Mechanic D 1969 *Mental Health and Social Policy.* Prentice-Hall, Englewood Cliffs, New Jersey.

Menuck MN & Seeman MV 1985 *New Perspectives in Schizophrenia.* Collier Macmillan Ltd, London.

Parsons T 1952 *The Social System.* Tavistock, London.

Peplau HE 1952 *Interpersonal Relations in Nursing: A Conceptual Frame of Reference for Psychodynamic Nursing.* GP Putnam's Sons, New York.

Peplau HE 1960 Talking with patients. *American Journal of Nursing,* 62, 6: 964–966.

Peplau HE 1962 Interpersonal techniques: The crux of psychiatric nursing. *American Journal of Nursing,* 62, 6: 50–54.

Peplau HE 1968 Psychotherapeutic strategies. *Perspectives in Psychiatric Care,* 6, 6: 264–289.

Peplau HE 1978 Psychiatric nursing: Role of nurses and psychiatric nurses. *International Nursing Review,* 25, 2 (March/April): 41–47.

Peplau HE 1985 An evaluation method for corrected use of language. *Personal communication,* 25th November. Sherman Oaks, California.

Rayner E 1978 *Human Development: An Introduction to the Psychodynamics of Growth, Maturity and Ageing,* 2nd Ed. George Allen & Unwin Ltd, London.

Rogers C 1942 *Counselling and Psychotherapy.* Houghton Mifflin Co, Cambridge, New Jersey.

Roy C 1980 The Roy Adaptation model. In *Conceptual Models for Nursing Practice,* 2nd Ed, J Riehl & C Roy (Eds). Appleton-Century-Crofts, New York.

Scott RD 1973 The treatment barrier. *British Journal of Medical Psychology,* 46: 45.

Smith L 1986 Issues raised by the use of nursing models in psychiatry. *Nurse Education Today,* 6: 69–75.

Sullivan HS 1953 *The Interpersonal Theory of Psychiatry.* WW Norton & Co, New York.

Vaughn GE & Leff JP 1976 The influence of family and social factors on the course of psychiatric illness. *British Journal of Psychiatry,* 129: 125–137.

Vaughn GE, Snyder KS, Freeman W, Jones S, Falloon IRH & Lieberman RP 1982 Family factors in schizophrenic relapse: A replication. *Schizophrenia Bulletin,* 8: 425–426.

5

Care plan for a confused person, based on Roper's Activities of Living model

Mike Thomas

This chapter demonstrates that it may be necessary to elaborate one or more elements of a model so that it fits the reality of nursing.

In this instance, it was felt that psychological aspects of patient assessment were inadequately addressed by the Roper *et al.* (1980) assessment schedule, and a psychological profile was drawn up by ward staff and used in conjunction with the existing documentation.

Confusion

A major problem encountered when dealing with the confused elderly person is one of defining confusional states. Panchaud (1984) defined the condition as one that is 'characterised by memory defects, sensory and perceptual changes, and verbal and non-verbal communication impairments'. She stressed that the environment is an important element in the manifestation of confusion. Confusion is not considered an illness, or a diagnosis, but a sign of disturbance with a cluster of symptoms. The importance of the environmental element is also noted by Roberts (1976), who suggested that the quality of the environment, the capacity of the senses to respond and the state of brain function were important key elements in confusional states.

Chalmers (1980), reports that the word confusion is often used as a diagnostic term and this leads to a failure of accurate diagnosis and inappropriate treatment and management. The co-existence of multiple pathology and disability can cause difficulty in separating confusion as a symptom, rather than a diagnostic entity. Chalmers goes on to discuss the fact that a confusional state in the young person is termed delirium, whereas in the elderly it is labelled dementia, reflecting differences in speed of onset, cause and prognosis.

Hunt (1977), defines a confusional state as one that is characterised by memory disturbance, disorientation and a loss of practical skills. Restlessness, aggressive behaviour and occasionally hallucinatory experiences may also be present and the state may have multiple causes. Like Chalmers (1980), she points out that if an elderly 'confused person' is wrongly labelled a 'demented old person', a return to their normal home environment is impaired by the different interventions given. Likewise Issacs (1979), suggested that once the label 'senility' is given to an elderly confused person, then the health professionals no longer investigate other causes. The elderly confused person is more at risk of this type of labelling as dementia and senility are often used synonymously.

Wolanin and Phillips (1981), define a confusional state as 'the behaviour that care givers recognise as being deviant from those expected from the client in a certain place and at a certain time'. These deviant behaviours include disorientation of time and place, defects in the memory, inappropriate speech and incongruous ideas.

The causes of confusion are difficult to ascertain unless a careful approach is used in information gathering. In the elderly, confusional behaviour generally falls into one of two categories or conditions. According to Chalmers (1980), these are the toxic confusional state (sometimes referred to as the acute confusional state), and the organic confusional state (dementia). However he points out that these conditions can co-exist with multiple pathology and disability, which can create problems in diagnosing the cause of confusional behaviour.

The acute confusional state may be caused by a myriad of generalised illnesses such as chest or urinary infections, myocardial infarction and many types of metabolic disturbances including diabetes, dehydration or hypothermia. Change of environment or life events such as bereavement or financial problems can also precipitate a confusional episode. Treatment or management of the causes usually removes the confusion. As Chalmers (1980), has noted, sufferers may also have organic brain damage and the response to treatment of a confusional state may be complicated.

A chronic confusional state, or dementia, is a global deterioration which is persistent and may be due to secondary aspects of extracerebral disease such as cerebrovascular degeneration, or due to cerebral pathology developing. Post (1978), states that research into chronic confusional states has largely centred on those sufferers who were physically fit or had central nervous system abnormalities. The research has confirmed that pathological brain changes and mental deterioration occur together and are progressive, ending in death.

Using clinical assessments, it is possible to differentiate between the pre-senile conditions (Pick's disease, Alzheimer's disease and Jakob-Creutzfeldt syndrome) and arteriosclerotic dementia in a large number of sufferers. However, there appears to be some evidence to indicate that Alzheimer's disease and arteriosclerotic disorders can occur simultaneously. As much as 25% of cases have been found by Corsellis (1962) and studies by Blessed *et al.* (1968) and Roth (1971) have supported these findings.

Other research into the causation of Alzheimer's disease has indicated the relevance of genetic factors. In a review of selected studies, Post (1978) concluded that chromosome losses occur more often in cases of chronic confusional states when compared with a control group of elderly people. He goes on to suggest that individuals of low intelligence or from low social classes are often falsely considered to be in the early stages of a chronic confusional state.

Investigations carried out by Feinberg *et al.* (1967), using EEG patterns during sleep, have shown demonstrable differences between young and old subjects, especially a reduction in periods of REM (rapid eye-movement) sleep. This reduction is more noticeable in sufferers of chronic confusional states.

Hunt (1977) suggests that one way of differentiating between an acute confusional state and a chronic confusional state is to establish the length of time since the onset of acute symptoms. She comments that the nurse is in an excellent position to gain such information from the relatives and friends of the client. This view is supported by Panchaud (1984), who says that any information obtained in this way is important in nursing the confused person. She further comments that the success of this process rests on the quality of the interaction between the client, the nurse and the client's family.

Unless the interaction allows the client to express his needs fully, and the nurse uses her expertise to work towards a common plan of action, then both partners will experience a growing sense of bafflement and helplessness which, as Panchaud points out, leads to frustration, anger and anxiety. Post (1978) states that good nursing makes use of lucid periods to establish better communication with the client and to diminish his panic and anxiety. He goes on to suggest that, for the person with a chronic confusional state related to physical disorders and social deprivation, mental impairment may be partly reversible with appropriate physical and social measures. Cosin *et al.* (1958) and Brook *et al.* (1975) suggest that occupational and social therapy may help such clients to adjust, but that the therapies have to be constantly and continuously undertaken. Chalmers (1980) comments that some degree of withdrawal and sensory deprivation are frequently encountered in many people with chronic confusional states. He points out that more can be achieved by personal interest, involvement and stimulation by the carer than can be achieved by medication. This suggestion supports that of Hunt (1977), that treating a confused client as if they have all their faculties and using verbal and non-verbal techniques, will often encourage the client to act 'normally'.

Panchaud (1984) studied sensory, self-care and communication skills within a group of five confused elderly people. She found that none of them perceived themselves as confused (although she observed one subject once put her hand to her head). She found no common pattern of memory loss, each subject having their own individual pattern. All the subjects had speech problems, which made interaction difficult and demanding. She concluded that the dominant need of the confused person was to remain 'spiritually alive', that is, to understand and shape reality, however difficult it becomes. The nurse's role is to respond to the client's communication needs, and the focus of all nursing activities should be on 'establishing and maintaining meaningful interaction between the client and his environment'. Panchaud (1984) also states that by using the relationship the nurse can assist the client to shape reality and retain a sense of identity. In return the client helps the nurse to develop expertise and skills, and gives value and strength to the professional self. An exchange can therefore exist which makes the relationship meaningful for both parties.

Selection of model

A study based on the Roper model (1976) of assessment was carried out with a client at a psychiatric unit catering specifically for the confused elderly people within Greater Manchester, during the Spring of 1986. The basis for choosing the model was centred on Roper's attempts to bring together a variety of insights from the physiological, psychological and nursing sciences to plan the nursing care of a client. Sundeen et al. (1981) commented that the nurse should 'always understand and have knowledge of the biological, physical and behavioural sciences to provide herself with a theoretical base for collecting data ... because this is the basis for implementing care'.

The research into confusional states indicates that a complex and delicate interaction occurs between physiological, psychological and environ-

mental conditions. The nurse should have insight into these interactions in order to assess, plan and implement adequate care with the confused person. According to Roper's model, one of the better ways of understanding human behaviour is in terms of the activities that humans perform. She identified specific activities of daily living which required assessment when formulating and implementing the nursing process approach. This model was subsequently elaborated by Roper et al. (1980).

The ward team decided to assess the confused person's ability to carry out independent activities of living in response to their own particular individual needs. This was in order to formulate and implement a plan of care to maintain the client's independence. Roper et al. (1980) identify factors which call for nursing intervention, these being disability, disturbed physiology, pathological and degenerative tissue changes, accidents, infections and effects arising from a person's physical, psychological or social environment. They comment that old age may call for nursing interventions related to particular activities at this stage of life, which can only be accomplished with the help of others. It was expected that assessment using the Roper AL framework would be completed within forty-eight hours of admission to the unit, and care plans implemented by then.

The assessment profile differs from that described by Roper et al. (1980). The documentation had been in use prior to the author's arrival on the ward, and had been modified when the ward was implementing the nursing process. During this modification, it had been suggested that 'working and playing' was a less significant AL than 'worshipping', and the latter had been substituted on the ward stationery. Since the work carried out for this chapter and the ensuing discussion, the assessment documentation has been modified again to include 'working and playing'. It is also recognised that former occupation and recreational activities form a relevant part of assessing and implementing care.

Patient assessment

Betty, a 75-year-old woman, was chosen as typical of the clients in the unit, since she manifested the effects of physiological disorder on her psychological state producing behaviour open to misinterpretation. She was admitted to the ward for a two-week assessment period after a domiciliary visit by the consultant geriatrician. Her home was an elderly people's residence near the hospital, where she had lived for the past five years. Over four weeks, her behaviour had drastically altered. She began to wander at night, was aggressive (both verbally and physically) on approaching other people and mistakenly thought that other people were relatives or friends from her past. Her GP had prescribed temazepam, which is indicated for insomnia. The medication had little effect except to cause drowsiness in the mornings.

Immediately on admission the assessment shown in Fig. 5.1 was completed. Betty appeared cheerful and lucid during questioning, although her short-term memory was poor. She was also disorientated as to her whereabouts and the time. She was continent, although understandably she needed directing to the toilet at first. Mobility and dexterity were good and she took adequate diet and fluids. The night staff reported that she slept soundly throughout the night.

Within 48 hours of admission Betty was observed to be experiencing hallucinations, both auditory and visual, during the night. Urinalysis had indicated a urinary tract infection at this time and a course of antibiotics was prescribed. Nursing care for the problem was implemented. Her physical condition continued to deteriorate and an assessment (Fig. 5.2) of her psychological state was completed by the nursing team. This was an

Fig. 5.1 Assessment of activities of living 1

Usual routines: what he/she can and cannot do independently Betty – Roper assessment one.	Date: Patient's problems (actual/potential) (p) = potential
Maintaining a safe environment	Appears disorientated to ward environment: potential hazard if she wanders at night, recent history of night wandering.
Communicating	Communicates well verbally. Short-term memory appears poor, and she requires prompting to answer questions regarding recent events. Full assessment required.
Breathing	Breathing normally.
Eating and drinking	Nutritious diet and fluids taken without any problems. No dislikes or preferences expressed. Has good social skills at meal times.
Eliminating	Betty is continent, however she requires guidance to the toilet as she is not familiar with the ward layout.
Personal cleansing and dressing	Dresses neatly and appropriately. Good standard of personal hygiene maintained.
Controlling body temperature	Maintains adequate body temperature, but recent history of night wandering is a potential problem.
Expressing sexuality	Appears aware of her appearance and behaves appropriately in social situations. Likes to put her make-up on prior to breakfast.
Mobilising	Mobilising well and has free movement of all limbs and joints. Requiring orientation to ward environment.
Sleeping	Sleeping well throughout the night, but prior to admission was observed to be wandering during the night.
Dying	Did not discuss aspects of mortality and illness when topic was tentatively approached.
Worship	States she is a non-practising Christian. Baptised in the Roman Catholic Church.

Fig. 5.2   Psychological assessment 1

Intellect Makes her needs known clearly, understands others, understands and responds well during conversation. Appears confused at times but has long periods of lucidity.
Emotion Appears cheerful, humorous and pleasant when involved in conversation. However Betty can become very agitated and distressed when she is experiencing hallucinations.
Volition Expresses her own wishes assertively but occasionally becomes confused when presented with several choices, or not being allowed enough time to reply to questions.
Orientation Disorientated in time and place, but recognises members of her family quite clearly.
Memory Short-term memory appears very poor and she needs constant reminders. She appears to be 'living in the past' and clearly recalls childhood experiences.

attempt to compare her mental state now she was physically unwell with her state on admission in order to decide whether she was deteriorating psychologically as well as physically. This involved measuring her intellectual abilities such as reaction time to verbal stimuli, clarity of thought, and complexity of thought. Also measured were her emotional state, (whether elated, anxious, suspicious, labile or appropriate); her volition, (whether passive or assertive); orientation to time, place and persons, and both her long- and short-term memory.

These measurements were collected by using both formal and informal methods. The formal methods involved asking such questions as her name, address, date, time and year. Informal methods included conversation, observation and participating in ward activities with Betty. The psychological assessment was then used with a reassessment (Fig. 5.3) using the Roper profile to decide the plan of care. The nursing team felt that the Roper profile was inadequate in gaining a deeper understanding of Betty's mental condition, and it was this reason which prompted the use of

the psychological profile in conjunction with Roper's.

Roper (1986) has stated that psychiatric nurses should develop the model as necessary, especially with regard to aspects of communication, to facilitate its use in psychiatric nursing. The approach used in assessing Betty's needs is therefore supported by Roper.

The plan of care included the administration of prescribed medication – haloperidol – for the control of behavioural disturbances. However, it became apparent that Betty was experiencing difficulty in maintaining her daily living activities and her level of dependence on nursing staff was increasing. It was decided when formulating a care plan (Fig. 5.4) to follow Roper's et al. (1980) advice that any nursing activity taken on Betty's behalf should be communicated to her. She was to be informed that such intervention was necessary but transient, until her independence could be regained.

During nursing interventions it was noted that Betty appeared to be breathing erratically although she stated that she felt fine and was in no distress. However, a physical examination was performed and a chest infection diagnosed; antibiotic therapy was prescribed. Based on the information that Betty now had a chest infection an evaluation of the care dealing with her psychological problems was carried out. It was decided that the planned nursing intervention was not achieving the specific goal, due to Betty's inability to respond to specific nursing interventions. Betty was reassessed and a new care plan was formulated (Figs 5.5 and 5.6). This involved implementing care to deal initially with physical problems. The short-term goals involved interaction with a confused, frail, bed-bound lady, the long-term objectives involved implementing care to help Betty be free of a chest infection. On physical recovery, a further assessment was to be carried out to determine her psychological state (Figs 5.7 and 5.8).

The Roper assessment profile showed how virtually all activities of living were affected, with communication difficulties being especially severe. As Hunt (1977) stated, this led to increased problems in dealing with the anxieties, frustrations and irritations experienced by Betty.

Fig. 5.3 Assessment of activities of living 2

Usual routines: what he/she can and cannot do independently Betty – Roper assessment two.	Date: Patient's problems (actual/potential) (p) = potential
Maintaining a safe environment	Constantly wanders around the ward. Potential hazard due to disorientation.
Communicating	Possibility that Betty is experiencing hallucinations, both visual and auditory. These are creating difficulties with communication.
Breathing	Breathing normally.
Eating and drinking	Continues to maintain a good dietary intake, however she is disturbing other residents who share her table by being abusive to unseen persons.
Eliminating	Occasionally incontinent of urine due to inability to find ward toilet.
Personal cleansing and dressing	Continues to dress neatly and appropriately, independent of nursing assistance.
Controlling body temperature	Maintains adequate body temperature and dresses appropriately.
Expressing sexuality	No change from previous assessment.
Mobilising	No change from previous assessment.
Sleeping	Experiencing disturbed sleep pattern. Shouting abuse at unseen persons.
Dying	No change from previous assessment.
Worship	No change from previous assessment.

Although some degree of impairment was noted when Betty initially entered the unit, she still maintained the ability to cater for most of her daily needs. As her condition became worse her independence became severely compromised, with more and more tasks being undertaken by the nursing team. Her ability to maintain a sense of reality, which Panchaud (1984) stressed as important for the confused person, was under threat. This was due to the severe communication problems encountered when trying to establish a therapeutic relationship between Betty and the care team.

Roper *et al.* (1980) state that not all individuals have the potential to be independent in all activities of daily living, but the goal should still be 'optimal independence' for each AL by carrying out an individualised care programme. Throughout Betty's illness, individual acts, no matter how small, were encouraged. Within two weeks her condition had substantially improved and an evaluation of her care plan showed that set objectives had been reached, both long-term and short-term goals.

Sundeen *et al.* (1981) and Roper *et al.* (1980) discuss the continuous evaluation of the care given to measure its effectiveness. Re-assessment would give a comparison between the original assessment to decide new, or different, nursing interventions. The haloperidol medication had been discontinued during Betty's illness and a psychological assessment (Fig. 5.8) was again carried out to ascertain whether she now required this. However, the new assessment did not record any indications of psychosis, although poor memory and some degree of disorientation were still apparent. A new plan of care was therefore implemented which involved encouraging independence and withdrawing nursing intervention dealing with Betty's AL needs.

The programme involved encouraging Betty to rely less on the hospital institution and staff, so as to enable her to return to the elderly people's home. It was hoped that further rehabilitative help would be given there. Betty now became involved in devising her own care plan and participated in evaluation. It was felt that she was prepared for her return to her

Fig. 5.4   Care plans 1 and 2

Name:	Betty			Ward		
Start date	Problem No. 1	Objective	Plan	Imple-mentation day/time	Evalu-ation day	Stop date and signature
8.4.86	*Actual:* Betty is experiencing auditory and visual hallucinations. These are disrupting her ability to cater for her daily needs.	Betty to cater for her daily needs independently.	1 Use distraction when Betty is observed to be experiencing hallucinations. Engage in conversation. 2 Observe and report effects of distraction. 3 Observe and report situation in which hallucinations occur. 4 Give prescribed medication. Observe and report effects.	9.4.86	15.4.86	15.4.86

Name:	Betty			Ward		
Start date	Problem No. 2	Objective	Plan	Imple-mentation day/time	Evalu-ation day	Stop date and signature
8.4.86	*Actual:* Social interaction is deteriorating.	Betty to maintain adequate social interactions. She will: – participate in group activities – take part in conversation.	1 Involve Betty in group conversations. 2 Involve Betty in group tasks. Encourage participation and assertion. 3 Engage in one-to-one conversation. Use prompting, focusing and concreteness. 4 Encourage independence at all times. Reinforce acts of independence.	9.4.86	15.4.86	15.4.86

Fig. 5.5   Assessment of activities of living 3

Usual routines: what he/she can and cannot do independently Betty – Roper assessment three.	Date: Patient's problems (actual/potential) (p) = potential
Maintaining a safe environment	Not mobilising due to chest infection. Unable to perform any activity of living unaided.
Communicating	Continues to experience sensory disturbances which are creating difficulties with communication.
Breathing	Has difficulty breathing at present due to chest congestion. Requires the aid of a suction machine at times to clear her mouth and throat.
Eating and drinking	Dietary intake deteriorating, requires a lot of prompting and encouragement even to maintain adequate fluid intake. Occasionally requires the help of a nurse to spoon-feed her which may lead to loss of dignity and self-esteem.
Eliminating	Requires the use of the commode hourly due to urinary incontinence, however Betty does ask for the commode when she wants to pass faeces.
Personal cleansing and dressing	Requires full nursing help to maintain hygiene. Requires a bed-bath daily due to profuse perspiration. Requires mouthwash regularly to maintain clean mouth.
Controlling body temperature	Experiencing high temperatures due to chest infection, requires tepid sponging and a fan at times. Potential problems may occur due to inadequate fluid intake.
Expressing sexuality	Betty is aware of her appearance but now requires assistance to dress appropriately and she is no longer wearing any make-up. She 'doesn't want to be bothered'.
Mobilising	Betty is not mobilising at all at the moment. She requires the help of two nurses to assist her from her bed to the commode.
Sleeping	Sleep pattern very disturbed. She is at present alternating between drowsiness and agitation.
Dying	Aware she is not 'herself' at present but cannot say why. Betty's family need support and comfort. They are staying at her bedside whilst she is ill.
Worship	Family will ask the staff if they feel a priest is required. They require information about her condition.

home when an evaluation of her care occurred two weeks after recovering from her chest infection. She expressed a wish to return there and believed she was ready for a less dependent environment. She participated in the multidisciplinary meeting which discussed her period in the unit and she was discharged the following day.

Evaluation and conclusion

On evaluating the effects of the Roper assessment in the care of Betty, several aspects were noted. It was felt that the frequent evaluation and re-assessments using the AL profile gave good indicators of the effects of nursing care given, and illustrated the different measures required in order to meet Betty's individual needs. The essentially dynamic nature of such an approach was observed through the various types of interventions required. However, such an approach can be demonstrated with any nursing model used within the nursing process approach to care.

One notable aspect of using the AL model when caring for Betty was the fact that her chest condition was initially investigated due to the

Fig. 5.6   Care plan 3

Name: Betty				Ward		
Start date	**Problem No. 3**	**Objective**	**Plan**	**Imple-mentation day/time**	**Evalu-ation day**	**Stop date and signature**
15.4.86	*Actual:* Breathlessness and copious secretions due to chest infection. Unable to perform ALs without assistance. Potential problems: skin lesions immobility due to bed rest.	1 Betty to be free of chest infection. 2 To cater for her needs independently.	1 Two-hourly position change.	15.4.86	Daily	28.4.86
			2 Observe and report skin condition.	15.4.86	Daily	28.4.86
			3 Nurse in upright position.	15.4.86	Daily	28.4.86
			4 Encourage 200 ml fluid hourly. Maintain fluid chart, and four-hourly TPR chart.	15.4.86	Daily	28.4.86
			5 Assist onto commode two-hourly.	15.4.86	Daily	28.4.86
			6 Converse with Betty while giving care – reorientate each time. Mobilise gradually: chair 22/4; walk 25/4.	15.4.86 22.4.86 25.4.86	Daily 25.4.86	28.4.86 28.4.86
			7 Encourage all acts of independence.	22.4.86	Daily	28.4.86
			8 Discuss progress with relatives.			

interaction and observation of a member of the nursing team: the assessment profile had recorded no difficulties or potential difficulties with her breathing. Betty herself stated that she felt fine and was not distressed. The Roper profile had not helped in the actual detection of Betty's chest condition, and it may be that the assessment would have to have been carried out daily, which is clearly not feasible and may induce in the nurse a form of nursing which would not involve other insights or considerations.

Although implementation of the activities of living framework appears to be workable, certain aspects which are of particular relevance to psychiatric nurses, and the care of elderly confused people, are lacking. The importance of a full assessment involving intellect, affect, volition, memory and orientation cannot be understated when attempting to plan the nursing care of the confused elderly person. Sensory disturbances, such as hallucinations, also need to be identified correctly if a therapeutic relationship is to develop. Consequently a psychological assessment profile needed to be designed by the nursing team, and

Fig. 5.7 Assessment of activities of living 4

Usual routines: what he/she can and cannot do independently Betty – Roper assessment four.	Date: Patient's problems (actual/potential) (p) = potential
Maintaining a safe environment	Mobilising around the ward but remains disorientated to ward layout. She is recovering from a chest infection and consequently becomes very tired quickly.
Communicating	Communicating her needs well. Betty's short-term memory continues to be poor and she requires prompting to recall recent events.
Breathing	Recovering from a chest infection, breathing without difficulty.
Eating and drinking	Betty is now taking a very good diet and fluids. Her social skills are good when she eats her meals with other residents.
Eliminating	Continent when shown location of the toilets.
Personal cleansing and dressing	Dresses neatly and appropriately, maintains her own standard of hygiene, no longer requires nursing assistance.
Controlling body temperature	Maintaining adequate body temperature, but this requires monitoring due to her recent illness.
Expressing sexuality	Aware of her appearance, dresses appropriately and behaves appropriately in social interactions. Seeing to her own make-up.
Mobilising	Mobilising freely around the ward, however she requires reminders to ensure she takes adequate rest periods.
Sleeping	Sleep pattern appears good, sleeping well throughout the night.
Dying	Betty jokes about the subject of death and dying when it is raised in conversation. She's 'too young to go yet'. Shows no insight into her recent illness.
Worship	States she is a non-practising Christian, baptised into the Roman Catholic Church.

then used with the Roper model. In this area of immense importance to psychiatric nursing the Roper model was considered inadequate by the nursing team.

Aggleton and Chalmers (1985) on analysing the Roper model, found that some activities identified by Roper *et al.* (1980) varied depending on the age of the client, the young and old being less independent in their performance of daily living activities. Also, as previously stated, Roper *et al.* (1980) comment that old age may call for nursing intervention related to particular activities at this stage of life, which can only be accomplished with the help of others. Difficulty may be encountered when assessing activities of living with individuals who experience chronic confusional states as there will be a continuous impairment of their ability to cater for their needs. The inability to cope with daily living tasks alone, however, does not take away the intrinsic 'individuality' of the person. There is a possibility that nurses using the Roper profile may lose sight of an individual's identity and worth because they cannot cope with daily living activities. Again the psychological needs of the individual, such as security, assertive, social and recreational needs are not fully addressed. A behaviourist dimension is implied, based on observable activities to cater for daily needs. Individuality, in the full sense of the word, was not considered to be adequately met when using the Roper model with the elderly confused person. Such considerations when using the AL approach to care have been discussed by Bowell (1986), who found that the Roper model tended to stress the physical aspects of care when

Fig. 5.8   Psychological assessment 2

Intellect   Makes her needs known clearly and is lucid during interactions. However she requires prompting at times as she forgets the thread of the conversation.
Emotion   Very cheerful and humorous when in conversation, expresses her emotions freely and interacts well with other residents on the ward. No agitation or anxiety observed.
Volition   Asserts herself and makes her wishes known. Requires time to respond to questions at times. Helping other residents at times.
Orientation   Remains disorientated to the ward environment, states she wants to go home. Recognises members of her family and staff on the ward. Requires reminders as to the date and time.
Memory   Short-term memory continues to be poor at times, requires prompting and reminders.   Long-term memory remains very good, no longer believes she is a young woman or that she is working, still recalls past experiences with clarity.

used in nursing individuals in isolation wards. In evaluating the nursing care of a patient in an isolation ward, she concluded that the Roper model was 'inadequate' in meeting non-physical needs.

In order to evaluate the Roper model a team meeting was held to discuss its use. Relatives and nurse learners were interviewed in an informal atmosphere to ascertain views and the subject raised in a multidisciplinary meeting. All involved expressed enthusiasm for such an approach, comments including the fact that communication was increased with the client, although the speaker admitted this was due to the psychological assessment being used with the Roper profile. Some members of the nursing team felt that the use of the model assisted in teaching nurse learners. By having specific care objectives it became easier to explain the rationales for rehabilitative techniques dealing with aspects of daily living. One member of the medical team commented that the Roper profile, in conjunction with the psychological assessment, helped in the diagnosis of specific daily needs.

Having twice-weekly staff meetings to discuss the Roper model and its implementation allowed worries and misgivings about the profile to be raised, and problems to be dealt with on a team basis. One member of the team speculated whether the model may be difficult to use when applied on a ward new to the nursing process itself, and whether inexperience in use would create confusion in setting objectives in Betty's care. The learners supported this view, stating that working with staff knowledgeable in the use of the model made it seem 'simpler to understand' and made them feel less insecure when implementing care. It was felt that a firm knowledge base in the use of the nursing process was an important prerequisite before the models could be used.

Problems regarding the limited emphasis on 'individuality' in the model and its implications for psychiatric care arose as the care of Betty progressed. The difficulty in assessing the confusional state was overcome by adding a psychological profile to the Roper assessment. In these aspects of individuality, the Roper model was considered inappropriate when used alone, particularly when nursing a confused elderly person.

References

Aggleton P & Chalmers C 1985   Models and theories 7. *Nursing Times*, **81**, 3: 33–35.

Blessed G, Tomlinson BE & Roth M 1968   The association between quantitative measures of dementia and of senile changes in cerebral grey matter of elderly subjects. *British Journal of Psychiatry*, **114**: 797–812.

Bowell E 1986   Nursing the isolated patient. *Nursing Times*, **82**, 38: 72–81.

Brocklehurst JC 1978   *Textbook of Geriatric Medicine and Gerontology*, 2nd Ed. Churchill Livingstone, Edinburgh.

Brook P, Degun G & Mather M 1975   Reality orientation: A therapy for psychogeriatric patients. *British Journal of Psychiatry*, **127**: 42–45.

Chalmers GL 1980   *Caring for the Elderly Sick*. Pitman Medical Ltd, Kent.

Corsellis JAN 1962   *Mental Illness and the Ageing Brain*. Oxford University Press, London.

Cosin LZ, Mort M, Post F, Westropp C & Williams M 1958   Experimental treatment of persistent senile confusion. *International Journal of Social Psychiatry*, **4**: 24–42.

Feinberg I, Koresko RL & Heller N 1967   EEG sleep patterns as a function of normal and pathological ageing in man. *Journal of Psychology*, **5**: 107–144.

Feinberg I & Carlson VR 1968   Sleep variables as a

function of age in man. *Archives of General Psychiatry*, 18: 239–250.

Hunt P 1977 Confusion in the elderly. *Nursing Times*, 73: 1928–1929.

Issacs B 1979 Don't bother – she won't notice. *Nursing Mirror*, 149, 18: 24–25.

Kay DWK & Walk A 1971 *Recent Developments in Psycho-geriatrics*. RMPA, Kent.

Panchaud CL 1984 *An investigation into confusion*. Unpublished MSc Thesis, University of Manchester.

Post F 1978 Psychiatric disorders. In *Textbook of Geriatric Medicine*, 2nd Ed, JC Brocklehurst (Ed). Churchill Livingstone, Edinburgh.

Roberts SL 1976 Behavioural concepts and the critically ill patient. *Journal of Advanced Nursing*, 7: 549–554.

Roper N 1976 *Clinical Experience in Nurse Education*. Churchill Livingstone, Edinburgh.

Roper N 1986 From *Nursing Models Conference*. Eastbourne.

Roper N, Logan W & Tierney A 1980 *The Elements of Nursing*. Churchill Livingstone, Edinburgh.

Roth M 1971 Classification and aetiology in mental disorders of old age: Some recent developments. In *Recent Developments in Psycho-geriatrics*, DWK Kay & A Walk (Eds). RMPA, Kent.

Sundeen SJ, Stuart GW, Rankin ED & Cohen S 1981 *Nurse–Client Interaction – Implementing the Nursing Process*, 2nd Ed. CV Mosby Co, St Louis.

Wolanin MO & Phillips LF 1981 *Confusion – Prevention and Care*. CV Mosby Co, St Louis.

6

Care plan for a suspicious person, using Roy's Adaptation model

Meg Miller

Systems-based models of nursing, such as Roy's (1976) Adaptation model, are often criticised as being reductionist and detracting from a holistic view of the person.

In this chapter, the suspicion of Colin, a 32-year-old married man, centres on two problems identified on assessment. However, the care plan shows how a holistic approach is reflected in the nursing action which recognises that although the two problems are recorded separately, they are interrelated.

The discussion of suspicion identifies the variety of theoretical underpinnings to the medical view of the condition, and the main nursing task of developing trust is demonstrated throughout the care plan.

Suspiciousness

Suspiciousness, when associated with mental illness, is nearly always synonymous with paranoia. In this case study it is a symptom of low self-esteem in a person whose pre-morbid personality made him vulnerable to paranoid ideation when faced with traumatic life events. While low self-esteem may be attributable to depression, in this instance the psychiatric label was of little help in understanding the complexity of the person's suspiciousness.

Sociological theory

Some theories of paranoia relate to this case. Paranoid symptoms may be attributable to both social and personality disintegrations (Post, 1982).

Some old but nevertheless relevant work by American sociologists after the Second World War suggested that paranoid symptoms resulted directly from attitudes towards self. Lemert (1951) describes the 'symbolic process' by which the individual distorts incoming communications in an attempt to marry up the extreme divergence between his own and others' attitudes towards him. The rejection of self is then accompanied by the rejection of others who are 'reciprocal points of reference for the intolerable subjective definitions of the self'. The concept of 'pseudocommunity' is described as the unreal world within which the paranoid person believes himself to exist.

> The pseudocommunity grows in clarity and sinister quality, being progressively expanded to include new activities and new personnel until the threat it represents reaches a crucial stage. At this point overt defensive or vindictive behaviour bursts forth which antagonises others and provokes counteraggressions which become the final verification of the deviant's fears and suspicions.
>
> (Lemert, 1951)

The behaviour which 'bursts forth' is likely to be perceived as deviant by those who witness it, and the sudden onset of paranoid ideas is likely to be associated with a specific problem or trauma.

> Contact with the patient is well preserved and the ideas are anchored in real, if idiosyncratically described, conflicts.
>
> (Post, 1982)

The development of such a personality may often be rooted in the behaviour of the individual's father in childhood. Studies have shown the families of paranoiacs to be 'authoritarian, demanding, harsh and cruel' (Kolb, 1977). The father is controlling and hostile, fostering in the child a poor self-image, fear, anxiety and feelings of inadequacy, and submission towards the father usually stems from the individual's longing to be loved (Tousley, 1984).

Psychodynamic theory

Freud (1911) asserted that the paranoiac has never developed his libidinal energy into external objects and has therefore stuck at the narcissistic stage.

Klein (1964) describes the 'paranoid position' of the infant, who fixes both good and bad feelings in his mother but fears that his bad feelings, for example greed and anger, may destroy the very object who makes him feel good. His only defence is projection – disowning his bad feelings and externalising them, thereby creating the sense of persecution of himself (Klein, 1964).

Interpersonal theory

Sullivan (1953) on the other hand attributes paranoid behaviour to learnt attitudes. He claims that when a child learns to maintain his self-esteem by belittling others, he does not learn to evaluate personal worth, neither his own nor others' (Tousley, 1984).

It is generally accepted that a significant aspect of the psychiatric nurse's role is that of her personal relationships with patients, and that this plays a substantial part in the nurse's contribution to therapy (Towell, 1975). In his study of psychiatric nursing practice, Towell (1975) found that by the end of their first year most nurses in training strongly agreed that 'the kind of relationship psychiatric nurses form with their patients can be an extremely important factor in the treatment of the patient's illness'. However, Altschul (1972) found that there was a lack of any treatment ideology or theoretical basis to nurses' contact with patients and the content of their interactions. She concluded that the probable cause is that 'nurses do not have any identifiable perspective to guide them in their dealings with problematic situations'.

The care plan therefore needs to reflect an attitude to nursing intervention that, while the therapeutic element may be the time spent with the patient talking about himself, there should be a clearly defined and attainable goal towards which both nurse and patient direct their energies. It is important for the nurse to realise that suspiciousness serves a function – it protects the individual from a hostile environment and reduces the anxiety which results from feeling vulnerable. Patients may protect themselves from overwhelming emotion by isolating themselves and this can often increase their sense of alienation (Stuart and Sundeen, 1983).

The nursing aim with a suspicious patient is to foster a relationship in which he comes to demonstrate trust in her. Meize-Grochowski (1984) defines five attributes of trust:

1 attitude
2 reliability
3 confidentiality
4 relevance to time and place
5 fragility

resulting in the following definition:

> Trust is an attitude bound to time and space in which one relies with confidence on someone or something. Trust is further characterised by its fragility.
>
> (Meize-Grochowski, 1984)

In other words, the individual who trusts someone or something must have experience of situations in which that trust could be broken but was not. Even so, the trust is easily broken and less easily re-established. In the case of a person with a generally suspicious personality, the nurse must strive to be honest, reliable and trustworthy (the latter having been tested over time), and be comfortable with continual self-analysis in order to discuss with the patient his progress towards being a trusting person (Stuart and Sundeen, 1983).

Thus the nurse forms part of the patient's social environment. Through constancy of input in the face of testing behaviour from the patient, the latter is encouraged to respond in a positive way to this new social environment. Such a perspective on the situation relates to the model of nursing developed by Roy (1976). Positive adaptation – becoming a trusting person – is promoted by controlling the environmental stimuli (including the nurse) to which the patient responds as an adaptive system.

Roy's Adaptation model

Sister Callister Roy's model is based on general systems theory. A person's system may be perceived as those elements within a stated boundary with which he constantly interacts. Outside the boundary is the environment. Tension, stressors, strains and conflict arise within the system boundary, though there is constant input, throughput and output across the boundary. The system has a tendency to achieve equilibrium, or a 'steady-state' (Riehl and Roy, 1980). Figure 6.1 is an example of a person's system.

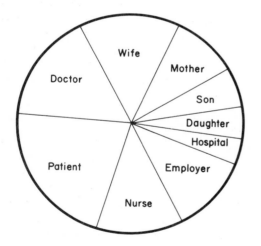

Fig. 6.1 Diagram of a patient's system, as implied in systems theory

Rationale for choice of model

The use of a model based on systems theory was favoured for the care of the individual under study, especially since he did not suffer from an organic complaint, but a functional disorder, with the inherent involvement of the person's environment. Roy's basic assumptions of a health–illness continuum and man being in constant interaction with his environment seemed most appropriate.

One reason for choosing Roy's model as opposed to another based on systems theory, such as King's (1971) theory for nursing, was that this was to be a care plan for a patient approaching discharge. As he had been in hospital for nearly two months, it was felt that his return to his home environment would necessitate considerable adaptation – to less dependence on the hospital, more responsibilities, more stress, return to work, and the probability of stigma from having been in a psychiatric hospital. The chosen time span for the care plan was two weeks. Any shorter time would scarcely show significant adaptive responses in a person with emotional difficulties, and this was the period of notice of discharge that the patient was given by the medical staff, though this was a vague rather than specific figure. In practice, however, the care plan was continued as the patient was not considered well enough to be discharged at the end of that period.

Outline and critique of Roy's Adaptation model

Roy bases her model on the assumption that man achieves equilibrium through adaptation in one or more subsystems, or adaptive modes, namely physiological, self-concept, role-mastery and interdependence. Other assumptions upon which her model is based are:

(a)   man is a biopsychosocial being;

(b)   man is in constant interaction with a changing environment;

(c)   biological, psychological and social facets are used by a person in coping with an ever-changing world;

(d)   life experience involves illness as well as health. Illness is not idiosyncratic;

(e)   adaptation to the environment is requisite in life;

(f)   stimuli in a person's environment guide the adaptation process;

(g)   positive adaptive responses result from stimuli within a person's repertoire of responses.

Adaptation is, therefore, essential for survival. Health and illness are both patterns of adaptive change, by which the organism seeks to retain its integrity (Levine, 1969).

Roy's model takes an holistic approach to the individual. Nursing requirements depend on a person's position on the health–illness continuum, which in turn depends on the person's response to his internal environment in interaction with the external environment. At the interface are the determinants of nursing intervention. Intervention is indicated if adaptation is inadequate for the person to maintain integrity without support. Roy identified man's adaptive level as being determined by three classes of stimuli:

1 **Focal** stimuli – those stimuli that immediately confront the person and to which he responds.
2 **Contextual** stimuli – those stimuli that contribute to the person's behaviour caused by the focal stimuli.
3 **Residual** stimuli – those stimuli that arise from the person's past experience.

(McFarlane, 1980.)

The ultimate aim of nursing using this model is to support and promote adaptation of the individual within the context of his own health–illness pattern, internal environment and stimuli available for use. Since the nurse actively participates in the person's environment, she is one of the contextual stimuli. She will introduce knowledge and skill into events that affect the person. Her intervention must be based not only on scientific knowledge, but on recognition of the individual's response that indicates the nature of the adaptation taking place. In other words the nurse must read correctly the message that the individual is communicating.

Critique of the model

One of the major strengths of this as a nursing model is the use made of the nurse–patient relationship, where the nurse may be seen as one of the contextual stimuli, and the patient is an active participant rather than passive receiver of care, and must be involved in decisions regarding this care. Without being prescriptive, therefore, it enables the nurse to identify her role in the patient's adapta-

tion. Personally, I found it difficult to distinguish between the focal stimulus and the presenting problem (not always the same), and the contextual stimuli and background information. However, this was not an insoluble problem. Interpretation of a model by its user must be acceptable, and indeed acts as validation of its worth as a nursing tool.

The model embodies the principles of individualised and holistic care. It specifies different levels of stimuli and therefore directs the nurse to make decisions on the most appropriate intervention for the individual rather than the same for all who share the same medical diagnosis. It is a strength of the model that illness is viewed as maladaptation rather than abnormality, and the model may therefore be used as appropriately for a healthy pregnant woman as for a very sick person. However, it might be difficult to persuade a person who is knocked down in the street that he was using maladaptive responses.

The acceptance of this model as a valuable contribution to nursing is not without its critics. The assumption that man has four adaptive modes is questioned by Roy herself (Riehl and Roy, 1980), while Galbreath (1980) questions the conceptualisation of an individual's wholeness and integrity based on the assumption that man is a biopsychosocial being. Altschul (1984) asserts that nurses 'cannot operate in the belief that a developmental approach is always right and proper (as is suggested by Roy)'. This reflects her disenchantment with the notion of there being any one theory of nursing 'in the absence of a consideration of the total system of beliefs and practices surrounding health care and of psychiatric health and disease in particular' (Altschul, 1984).

Finally, readers new to American nursing literature may experience difficulty understanding the language.

Patient history

Colin Bourne is a 32-year-old married man with two children, Gemma aged 8, and Mark aged 6. During his ten years of married life with his wife, Jean, there had been nothing remarkable about their daily routine.

He had worked hard at his job as a scaffolder, enjoying the physically strenuous element and the good feeling he got from doing a 'man's job'. He drew pleasure from his visits to the pub with the lads occasionally, yet loved his home life and wanted the best for his family. From working hard and doing as much overtime as he could, Colin had managed to secure a mortgage on a house of their own in Thornton Heath. This was situated in an up-and-coming area and Colin and Jean were thrilled to find a semi-detached, 3-bedroomed house that they could afford. It had needed some work to be done on it, but Colin was good with his hands and liked the idea of improving the house himself.

Colin and Jean didn't go out much. They occasionally had some friends round to supper, but it was difficult to get baby-sitters and anyway they needed the money for the house. Jean would have liked to go out more. She liked going to parties, and would have appreciated being invited to go to the pub with Colin once in a while, but Colin never asked. He had always been a bit edgy when she was with his friends. More than once he had actually accused her of flirting with them, and he had hit Jack one night when he had made a pass at her. Nevertheless, she had been content, Colin was a good husband, never treating her or the kids badly, and he worked hard to give them all the best of everything.

He was an attractive man. Clean-shaven, of medium height and build, with thick dark blond hair; he took a pride in his appearance, always dressing well and exercising regularly to keep his weight down. He could take as long as Jean to get ready on the rare occasions when they did go out, blow-drying his hair and pressing his jeans so they had neat creases down the front.

Colin's children loved him. He would always play with them when he got home from work and encouraged them with their homework. He had a thing about that. He always told them he wished he had been made to do his homework when he was at school as he might have got some O levels if he had worked harder.

Suddenly, in September 1985, he was made redundant. There had been no warning, just an announcement that the management did not have enough work to justify keeping them all in employment. Colin had been stunned. For the first time in their marriage he had cried in front of Jean. Why him? What had he done to deserve this? Had someone told the boss of the tools he had borrowed last month to do a job on the house? Jack maybe?

For two days Colin had taken to his bed. Then Jean had told him to pull himself together and that this was no way to behave. So he had got up, bathed and shaved and had felt better, but when Jack rang up to suggest they met in 'The Anchor' for a drink, he would not go.

As the days went by he felt less and less like going out. He did not like Jean going out either. The atmosphere between them became tense. They argued a lot. Jean nagged at him to at least get on with the house instead of lying around feeling sorry for himself. He knew he should but, well, he just couldn't get round to it. He even went to his GP who said he was depressed and gave him some pills. They didn't help. How could they? It was her who was the problem . . . harping on all the time . . . just waiting for an excuse to go out flirting herself around town. . . . Had to keep an eye on her . . . couldn't be sure what she was up to. . . . Heard her saying to the kids the other day that they might have to move if I didn't get a job. She's plotting to take them away from me, that's what it is. . . .

Admission to hospital

Colin was admitted to hospital via the Outpatients Department on 14th April, 1986. His admission was precipitated by his taking the children and leaving home without his wife's knowledge. He had been found by his wife's family and brought to hospital, with paranoid symptoms much in evidence. He was convinced his wife had been going to take the children and that she had been unfaithful to him on several occasions.

He accepted hospital admission voluntarily, saying he felt it would be best if he were away from home for a while. Although clean, tidy and well-dressed, he looked tired and preoccupied, and conversed little with his wife. He smoked continuously throughout the admission interview, and avoided all eye contact.

Mrs Bourne appeared concerned and quite

distressed. She left soon after Colin's arrival on the ward.

Having been seen by his doctor, Colin was prescribed a phenothiazine drug to control his psychotic symptoms and a drug to control side effects. A differential diagnosis was made of:

(a) paranoid reaction;
(b) depression;
(c) morbid jealousy.

Assessment

Roy identifies two distinct levels of assessment: the first being the classification of the person's behaviour into adaptive and maladaptive responses; the second being the formulation of a nursing diagnosis, and decision as to which of the relevant stimuli may be manipulated in an attempt to overcome difficulties the person is experiencing.

A guide to nursing assessment is offered in Fig. 6.2 as an aid to interviewing the person according to Roy's four adaptive modes. Figures 6.3 and 6.4 give Colin's initial assessment and problem identification within these guidelines, and Figs 6.5–6.7 show the care plans implemented.

Evaluation

Figure 6.8 shows excerpts from the daily notes as kept on Colin Bourne between 24th May and 2nd June, 1986. They stand as on-going evaluation which is summed up on the care plans. (All names used are fictitious.)

Critique of the model in use

The fact that the patient's condition deteriorated during the period in which the care plan was carried out does not detract from the appropriateness of the planned intervention. It would appear that the patient's condition would have deteriorated rapidly following his discharge, probably necessitating his readmission, and that the results of the nursing intervention and the time spent with Colin identifying his problems and setting goals with him, brought to the staff's notice the probability of there being major marital difficulties between the patient and his wife. It is also considered that this was a more significant factor in causing Colin's illness than his being unemployed, as was first thought.

An increase in the amount of disturbed behaviour on the ward highlighted one problem with regard to Roy's model. It is not simply the unfamiliar American terms but the abstract concepts that Roy refers to that make the framework difficult to understand. In a busy ward, where three nurses are on duty per shift for 20–26 patients, with only one of those a qualified RMN, it is likely that patient care will take priority over the writing of care plans. It is therefore unlikely that nurses will grapple with unfamiliar concepts in their endeavour to formulate a workable care plan. Hopefully, assessment, planning and evaluation all take place in the nurse's mind as she interacts with a patient. In an unduly disturbed ward, at best the nurses join in verbal consultation with each other regarding patients' care. This highlights the need for written care plans, but for a model to be used effectively, it must be simple, easily interpreted, and be embodied in the total nurse training curriculum.

The advantages of Roy's model in this study include the relative ease with which the team reached a nursing diagnosis for Colin. While a medical model is predominant, this is an elusive goal, unless of course it follows on directly from the treatment the patient is prescribed. For example, if a patient is sufficiently disturbed to require sedation, but lacks insight into this, the nursing diagnosis might be that he requires to be medicated against his will. Where the nursing assessment elicits perceptions of the individual's self-concept – how much in control of his destiny he believes he is, whether he can express anger, joy, sadness or hurt, or how accepting he is of his patient role – one enters realms of the person's experience that are rarely the concern of the psychiatrist, yet may contribute enormously to the person's psychopathology. With a medical diagnosis, the psychiatrist finds direction for his treatment of the patient. With a nursing diagnosis, nurse and patient together move in the direction of change, greater understanding of self, and growth. In the case of

Fig. 6.2   Guide to nursing assessment – to be used as an aid for interview

PSYCHOLOGICAL NEEDS	
Self-concept	
Physical self:	How does the person see himself? Does he like the way he looks? Does he believe it is important to look good? Does he express his individuality through his appearance? If so, what does he like to show the world through his appearance?
Personal self, *Moral ethical self:*	Is the person a worrier? If so, has he learnt this from his parents? Does he have faith in the worth of his own value system and attitudes? Does he often feel guilty? If so, about what sort of things?
Self-consistency and anxiety:	Does the person think he presents a consistent self-image? How does this compare with how he would like to be perceived? Does he feel anxious often? If so, about what sort of things? How does he express anxiety? What coping mechanisms does he use to overcome anxiety and how effective are they?
Self-ideal and expectancy *powerlessness:*	How does the person view himself as his own agent? Does he feel he has control over his destiny? What are his life expectations? How realistic are they? How does he cope with loss of control over his own daily life? i.e. does he adapt easily to hospital routine or does he resent it?
Interpersonal self:	Does the person have reasonable self-esteem? Does he like himself? Does he believe in his own worth? How assertive is he in getting what he wants? How does he portray himself in company? Does he express himself confidently or does he withdraw from company? Can he express anger, hurt, sadness, joy, love, triumph and pleasure? If so, how? Does he believe he has something to contribute to society? Does he believe he is interesting?
SOCIAL NEEDS	
Role-mastery:	How does the person accept the sick role? How does he feel about being a patient in a psychiatric hospital? Does he acknowledge his patient status? Does being a patient have implications for his other roles? Is he the breadwinner of the family? Might he lose his job? Is he unable to carry out his role as spouse, parent, lover, member of a group, club or team? How might his illness affect his ambitions, e.g. will it conflict with his job? How will his spouse or lover react to his having a psychiatric illness? Will it affect his plans for marriage or children?
Interdependence:	How does the person relate to staff? How does he express his needs? Does he use inappropriate behaviour, such as violence to himself or others, excessive demands, lack of sensitivity to other events, jealousy of nurses spending time with other patients? How does he relate to his relatives? Has he developed independence from his parents or parent figures? How does he relate to other patients? Is he well-liked or disliked? If disliked, does he have insight into this? Does he care about others around him? How does he show concern? Does he accept others' concern for him? Can he share? How does the person behave in public? Is he humorous or lacking sense of humour? Does he talk to strangers and if so, do they respond favourably? Is he aware of his effect on others? Does he reject kindness? Is he afraid of being rejected? If so, has he suffered rejection in the past?

Fig. 6.2 (continued)

PHYSIOLOGICAL NEEDS

Exercise and rest: Does the person have any problems ensuring adequate exercise and rest? Is he overactive? Is he motor-retarded? Does he sleep too much? Does he suffer from insomnia? Does he use night sedation?

Nutrition: Does the person have any problems maintaining an adequate diet? Is he overweight? Is he underweight? Has he lost or gained weight recently? Has he got a poor appetite at present? Has he an excessive appetite? Does he eat hospital food? Is he suspicious about food served up for him? Has he any special dietary needs?

Elimination: Does the person have any problems with elimination? Does he suffer from incontinence? Can he pass urine freely? Is urine free of blood, protein, sugar? Has he any problems with his bowels? Does he suffer from constipation? Does he use laxatives? Is he able to have sexual intercourse? If female, are there any problems with menstruation?

Fluids and electrolytes: Does the person drink enough? Does he suffer from oedema? Is he dehydrated?
Check weight.

Oxygen and circulation: Does the patient have any medical condition or history of same such as chronic bronchitis, heart failure, myocardial infarction or hypertension? Check blood pressure and pulse rate. Does the person smoke?

Regulation

Temperature: Is the person able to maintain a temperature within normal limits? Does he wear enough clothing? Does he wear too many clothes for the state of the weather? Does he have excessive baths? Does he dry himself properly afterwards? Does he wear shoes?

Senses: Does the person protect himself from injury? Is he a danger to himself? Does he suffer from any sensory deprivation, e.g. hearing or sight? If so, does he wear a hearing aid or spectacles? Does the person suffer pain? If so, from what cause? What does he normally do to control the pain?

Endocrine system: Does the person suffer from any endocrine disorder, e.g. diabetes? If so, how is it controlled? Does he receive any regular medication? If female, is she on the contraceptive pill?

Roy's model, this is a change or growth in the form of adaptation, suggesting active participation in the change process on the part of the patient/client/individual.

As this author sees it, this model is just one way in which nurse and patient can find mutual direction. In Colin's case, it was eminently suitable since it was as Colin approached discharge from hospital that the care plan was formulated. The focus of the plan was his adaptation to his home circumstances. However, another aspect of Colin's situation was his relationship with his wife. Since Roy views the person as an adaptive system in isolation within his environment it could be suggested that the interpersonal aspects of Colin's problem were not addressed. If it had been possible to think of the *couple* as an adaptive system, and nursing care had been directed to the two of them as a unit, then the difficulties which Colin experienced in adapting to home life may not have been so acute.

This suggests that different nursing models may be suitable at different times in a person's contact with a nurse, or in different environments such as at home or in hospital. While this is possible, it must not be presumed that there is only one 'right'

Fig. 6.3   First level assessment: data collection

Date: 23.5.86	Name: .... Colin Bourne ....

Adaptive Mode – Self-concept

Adaptive responses	Maladaptive responses
Physical self: Takes a pride in his appearance. Tidy and smartly dressed. Does not dress to create an impression. Believes appearance is not the only indication of what a person is like, but looking clean shows that one cares about oneself.	
Moral/ethical self: Does not consider himself a worrier, although tends to be pessimistic rather than optimistic.	Feels guilty about not being at home to help look after the children.
Self-consistency anxiety: Thinks he presents an image of a jovial, joking person when well. Could not keep this up when ill, but would like to regain this image.	Tends to withdraw and isolate himself when anxious. Expresses paranoid ideas about his relatives when more than one visits at a time.
Self-ideal and expectancy powerlessness: Feels in control of his daily activities. Finds it easy to approach staff if he needs help.	Worried that his being an inpatient of a psychiatric hospital will jeopardise his chances of getting a job – realistic worry.
Interpersonal self: Does not feel inferior as a result of being unemployed. Skilled at carpentry and general handyman work as well as at his occupation – scaffolding. Always attends ward groups and occupational therapy.	Used to have a lot of self-confidence, but now has a low self-esteem. Feels this has been taken away from him and put in someone else. Feels bad about his lack of literacy skills. Lacks confidence in socialising.

Adaptive Mode – Role Mastery

Plays with the children when he goes home.	Suspicious of his wife so has ceased sexual relations with her. His loss of job means he is no longer the breadwinner. He withdraws from socialising when the relatives visit because of his suspicions.

Adaptive Mode – Interdependence

Adaptive responses	Maladaptive responses
Relates well with staff and patients. Able to offer emotional support to other patients. Appreciates concern expressed for him and does not reject kindness. People warm to him as he tends to put on a happy face.	Suspicious of relatives. Withdraws from their company. Finds social occasions stressful. Rejection towards his wife due to his suspicions. 30.5.86 Expresses concern at the lack of nurses available now the ward is much busier. Psychotic ideas have increased, e.g. talks of his wife and her family plotting a conspiracy against him, as he did on admission.

Fig. 6.3   (continued)

Adaptive Mode – Physiological	
Exercise and rest: Sleeps for 6–7 hours each night with sedation.	Tends to spend a lot of time on his bed when he goes on leave. Not exercising as regularly as he did before coming into hospital. Restless last few nights, having nightmares and waking up with headaches.
Nutrition: Eats a well-balanced diet. Maintains normal healthy weight.	
Elimination: Passes urine without difficulty. Nothing abnormal in urine. Occasionally constipated but does not take laxatives.	
Fluids and electrolytes: Drinks 2 l per day.	Previous alcohol abuse. There may be a risk of his resorting to alcohol when anxious.
Oxygen and circulation: No dyspnoea. No evidence of palpitations or tachycardia when stressed.	Slight dizziness caused by antidepressants lowering his blood pressure. Smokes up to 20 cigarettes daily.
Temperature; senses; endocrine system: Nothing abnormal.	

model for any one situation. On the contrary, a nursing model is a tool to enable and facilitate nursing, rather than to constrain it. Only if viewed in this way will nursing models be a valuable contribution to nursing care.

Nursing the suspicious person – management and education implications

As previously stated, the therapeutic climate in nursing is arguably that of mutually agreed goals towards which nurse and patient direct their energies.

In many cases, the person may be unaware of his desires. In Colin's case for example, he may have wanted to leave his wife, but been unable to acknowledge this even to himself. He may therefore have been using defence mechanisms, such as denial and projection, and thus convinced himself that his wife was about to leave him. There is no quick, easy way for nurses or doctors to help this person to bring into his consciousness those things

he finds most difficult to accept. Unlike nursing the acutely ill patient where the essence of skilled nursing is to sense and supply his need, with patients who experience difficulties and disturbances in their relationships, the nurse's task is quite different. Here, her skills must lie in helping the person to face such problems as returning to home and work (Weddell, 1968). These skills may be learnt both in the classroom (Dietrich, 1978) and through practical experience. In Colin's case, they include fostering a relationship of trust, promoting self-esteem in the patient, and providing the milieu in which growth and change can occur.

Fostering a relationship of trust

By observing certain principles in her communication with the patient, the nurse may facilitate the development of his trust in her. Giving information freely to the patient, and if appropriate, relatives, with issues of confidentiality having been discussed early on in the relationship, will give the patient less real cause for suspicion, as will the nurse's refusal to participate in secrecy, a pattern of behaviour with which the family may have learnt to communicate.

Fig. 6.4   Second level assessment: problem identification

Date: 23.5.86			Name: Colin Bourne	

Patient's problem: Lack of self-confidence.

Stimuli			Nursing diagnosis	Stimuli to be manipulated
Focal	**Contextual**	**Residual**		
Change in life circumstances (redundancy)	(a) Colin's low self-esteem, and belief that this has been taken away from him and put in someone else. (b) People's view of themselves is strongly influenced by others' views. (c) Colin's poor literacy skills. (d) Colin's skills in working with his hands. (e) Availability of teacher to help with his literacy. (f) Ward groups and occupational therapy both of which he attends. (g) Takes care of his appearance.	(a) Colin's average IQ. (b) Lack of recognition of his skills by his parents when young.	Colin lacks self-confidence, probably largely because of his poor literacy skills and as a result of being made redundant. He has no confidence in socialising; he tends to drink quite a lot if out with friends, and when anxious.	Contextual stimuli (a) and (b). Later on (c) (d) and (f).

Patient's problem: Finding it difficult to go home on leave.

Stimuli			Nursing diagnosis	Stimuli to be manipulated
Focal	**Contextual**	**Residual**		
Fear of recurring suspiciousness.	(a) Discharge date set for 2 weeks. (b) Lives near enough to visit home frequently before then. (c) Returning to same circumstances as before his admission, i.e. to his home with wife and children. (d) Colin's increased awareness of his response to home visits being suspiciousness, namely expression of paranoid ideas about relatives; distrust of wife → no sexual relations; and withdrawal. (e) Colin's willingness to accept emotional support.	(a) Colin's perception of the man's role in the family being that of breadwinner, and guilt at not fulfilling this. (b) Colin's belief that his illness will be a stigma from now on. (c) Colin's history of turning to drink when anxious and depressed.	As Colin's discharge approaches, he is going on leave more often but is expressing suspicions about his wife's fidelity again. He tends to withdraw to his bed quite a lot when at home and is not having sexual relations with his wife. He is sleeping badly and gets headaches.	Focal stimulus. Contextual stimulus (d) and (e).

Fig. 6.5 Care plan 1

Date: 24.5.86			**Name:** Colin Bourne	
Problem	**Long-term target**	**Objectives**	**Nursing intervention**	**Evaluation** Date: 30.5.86
Lack of self-confidence. Low self-esteem.	To develop self-confidence.	By end of week 1: 1 Colin to identify specific aspects of himself that contribute to low self-esteem. 2 Colin to recognise those things he is good at and express something positive about himself to a nurse.	1 Provide opportunities for Colin to talk about times when he feels least positive about himself. 2 Encourage Colin to say something positive about himself, e.g. what he has achieved each day that he found difficult.	Objectives not achieved due to the disturbed ward atmosphere. (Added contextual stimulus: lack of time available for nurses to spend talking to Colin.)
Has difficulty spending long periods of time at home.	To adapt positively to his home environment.	By the end of week 1: 1 Colin to identify those situations that he finds difficult at home. 2 Colin to establish how he copes with difficult situations. 3 Colin to spend less time on his bed at home.	1 Discuss visits with Colin before and after he goes home. 2 Discuss visits with Mrs Bourne on Colin's return. 3 Provide Colin with opportunities to discuss his anxieties. 4 Ask Colin to note how long he spends on his bed each home visit.	1 Colin finds his relationship with his wife very stressful. 2 He rejects her physical approaches and becomes quiet and suspicious. 3 He spent some time alone in his room on his first visit, but stayed downstairs for the second visit.
Signature of nurse formulating care plan:				

Trust will also be promoted if the following are observed.

(a) Promises that are not within the nurse's control to keep are not made, for example, 'You will get better' or 'Of course your wife will visit'.

(b) Commitments made to the patient are followed through, for example, 'I'll come back and talk to you later'.

(c) Feelings that the patient may detect through the nurse's non-verbal communications are not denied if the converse is true, for example, 'No, I'm not angry'. The nurse can learn the skill of acknowledging feelings and communi-cating these to the patient without imputing blame. For example, 'Yes, I am angry. I feel angry whenever you suggest I am not acting in your best interests' is different from 'You make me angry with your false accusations'.

Promoting self-esteem

Having identified by means of a questionnaire, such as that outlined in *Human Needs and the Nursing Process* (Yura and Walsh, 1982), specific aspects of Colin's life that contributed to his poor self-esteem, it was decided to give him feedback on his achievements in those areas, since 'people's

Fig. 6.6   Care plan 2

Date: 30.5.86			Name: Colin Bourne	
Problem	**Long-term target**	**Objectives**	**Nursing intervention**	**Evaluation** Date: 2.6.86
Lack of self-confidence. Low self-esteem.	To develop self-confidence.	By the end of week-end: 1 Colin to identify specific aspects of himself that contribute to low self-esteem. 2 Colin to recognise his abilities and express something positive about himself to a nurse.	1 Give Colin questionnaire on self-esteem to complete. 2 Encourage Colin to say something positive about himself each day. Night nurse to approach him and ask how he has spent his day.	1 Results of questionnaire: Colin (a) does not feel in control of his life or health; (b) has a tendency to withdraw in social situations; (c) believes he has poor academic skills, e.g. literacy skills. 2 Expressed his achievement of a lot of progress while he has been here on 30.5.86. Not since.
Colin expresses psychotic ideas and says his relationship with his wife is breaking down.	Nurses to establish facts about marital disharmony.	By end of week 1: 1 Colin and Mrs Bourne to discuss their relationship in presence of nurse. 2 Colin and Mrs Bourne to give independence accounts of home leave. 3 Mrs Bourne will be aware of support available.	1 Ask Colin to keep a diary on next home visit. See Mrs Bourne on Colin's return. Compare accounts. 2 See Colin and Mrs Bourne together with Colin's doctor with a view to considering marital therapy. 3 See Mrs Bourne alone and allow her time to express her feelings.	**Evaluation date:** 6.6.86
Signature of nurse formulating care plan:				

views of themselves are strongly influenced by others' definition of them' (Jourard, 1974).

Yura and Walsh (1982) state

A review of the literature on self-esteem points to the importance of feedback from significant others in the development of self-esteem.

The approach was altered midway through the fortnight due to the added contextual stimulus of nurses' lack of availability to Colin since the ward had become disturbed. Driever (1976) identified low self-esteem behaviours using Roy's Adaptation model. Among the most common manifestations of low self-esteem were expression of feeling unable

Fig. 6.7 Care plan 3

Problem	Long-term target	Objectives	Nursing intervention	Evaluation Date: 10.6.86
Lacks confidence in himself especially in social situations and because of poor literacy skills.	To develop self-confidence.	By the end of week 2: 1 Colin to recognise his social skills. 2 Colin to be introduced to a teacher for literacy classes.	1 Give Colin verbal positive feedback when he contributes in ward groups. 2 Contact teacher in adolescent unit school.	

| Date: 2.6.86 | | | Name: Colin Bourne | |

Signature of nurse formulating care plan: ....

to confront difficulties, and expression of self-deprecation. It was therefore considered therapeutic for Colin to express something positive about himself each day. Since the evenings tended to be quieter and Colin tended to stay up late, it was decided that night nurses should encourage this behaviour by asking Colin what he had done each day. High self-esteem is associated with acceptance of responsibility for one's own life (Stuart and Sundeen, 1983). To engender that feeling of self-worth in another, the nurse needs not only to demonstrate her own belief in that person's worth, but also to help him to rely on personal feedback, for example achievements and recognition of positive attributes.

Coopersmith (1967) identified the types of experiences that promote self-esteem in the child.

1 Total or near total acceptance by parents.
2 Clearly defined and enforced limits.
3 Opportunities and latitude for individual action within defined limits.

Providing a therapeutic milieu

In an adult with low self-esteem, it would seem prudent to remember these when offering a therapeutic milieu. The person is then accepted at all times even if his behaviour is not, and the difference in this acceptance is clearly defined. Within defined limits, for example limits on display of aggression or sexual desires, the person is allowed to be autonomous, making his own decisions about what time to get up or go to bed; whether to attend group or occupational therapy; whether or not to be polite, or considerate of others, or to share. Such a milieu defies the nurse to be authoritarian, judgemental or custodial, or to see fit to impose a care plan on a patient without his involvement. For the nurse to provide such a milieu, she herself must have reasonable self-esteem.

If the nurse is uncomfortable with herself, her abilities, and her needs, then her chances of being able to interact therapeutically with clients are greatly reduced.

(Yura and Walsh, 1982)

This has implications for managers and educationalists, both of whom must in their turn respect the nurse's need for autonomy (both professional and in learning), but also assumes the nurse accepts responsibility for her own life and thus demands a commitment on the part of the nurse to developing self-awareness, and acceptance of her own accountability – both professionally and in learning.

Fig. 6.8   Nurses' progress notes on care plan interventions

Nursing interventions (from care plan)	Progress notes
24.5.86 (Colin has been seen by Dr Mayfield and may go home twice over the next four days.) Sit down with Colin and go through his new care plan with him.	Spent time with Colin and went over his new care plan with him. He became tearful twice during the conversation. He said it would take a long time for him to explain how this past year's events have brought him to this point and that it is largely to do with his relationship with his wife. Feels he needs to sit down and talk with her. Plans to go home on Saturday and knows that we will speak with his wife when he returns.
Approach Mrs Bourne and let her know we would like to talk to her about Colin's time at home.	Jean did not realise that her husband could go home twice over the weekend. Apparently Colin had not mentioned this to her. Will expect nurse to speak to her alone after Colin's next visit home. **D Shields**
25.5.86 Talk to Colin about his forthcoming home visit. Identify with him what was causing his anxiety.	Colin talked for a long time about his wife and a complex delusional system unfolded. His wife and family, he believes, are conning him and are involved in a conspiracy against him. He became very tearful. Says in the past his wife has refused to be touched or to sleep with him. He feels that his wife may still leave him, but is angry about this as he feels she is leaving having made money out of him. Colin's delusions seem to be interwoven with his feelings of inadequacy to make his wife happy. **B Feldman**
Night	No further delusional ideas expressed. Colin retired to bed around 11.30 pm. after watching TV. Slept rather poorly. **TNS**
26.5.86 pm Speak to Colin's wife when they return and also to Colin.	Jean said the visit went quite well. Nothing unusual happened. However, she felt Colin was quieter than usual. He spent some time alone in his room but did play games with the children. Colin said he found the evening quite tiring. Appeared subdued on return to the ward. Will go home again on Monday. **D Shields**
Night	Went for a walk during the evening. Later watched the late film on TV. Fairly good mood. Slept well. **TNS**
27.5.86 Provide Colin with the opportunity to discuss his anxieties.	Colin talked about his relationship with his wife and how it is breaking down. Feels he is now on the verge of ending the marriage. Thinks his mind is more in order now and he can think logically about the past. His home life is his main problem now as he feels he could go back to work. Still sees his wife as deceiving him and greedy. Hates going home. Says the house is no longer like home. **D Shields**

Fig. 6.8 (continued)

Nursing interventions (from care plan)	Progress notes
28.5.86 Discuss today's visit with Colin on his return and talk to Mrs Bourne about the visit.	Jean felt the visit had gone fairly well. Colin spent all day downstairs with the family. His brother-in-law and four children were there. Jean said there was only one thing that seemed strange to her. Colin said 'Do I smell or something? People seem a bit stand-offish.' Didn't have much time alone with him. Said how rejected she felt when she tried to cuddle him. Colin said the visit went fairly well, that he sat downstairs. He felt tense twice – it was the horse-racing that made him feel that way. Said it felt a bit more like home. Made no mention of people being stand-offish. **D Shields**
29.5.86	Colin attended the ward group and was quite supportive to the other patients. Superficially cheerful. No delusional ideas. **B Feldman**
30.5.86 am Assess Colin's mood as he is rather quiet and withdrawn.	Colin finds the noise and disruption caused by a disturbed patient hard to cope with. He awoke with a headache and describes feeling nervous and tense. Has been isolated in his room all morning and has complained of feeling unwell. **G Wilson**
Night Spend time with Colin. Encourage him to express something positive about himself.	Colin feels he has made a lot of progress while he has been here. **D Shields**
31.5.86 Spend some time with Colin. Encourage him to say something positive about himself.	Found Colin in the dormitory at 2.30 pm. He looked very low and admitted to feeling 'fed-up'. Feels uncomfortable on the ward at present. Says the atmosphere is different. **G Wilson**
1.6.86 Spend time with Colin allowing him to talk about whatever he likes. (He is isolating himself.)	Colin was reluctant to talk at first. Very suspicious of his wife. He is not sure whether to go home on Monday. When Jean visited he went to see his doctor. Jean was tearful, says she has been advised not to visit or let Colin go home at the weekend. Things very strained between Colin and Jean. **B Feldman**
Night	Colin remained on the ward for most of the evening but went out for a brief period. Rather unhappy and low in mood due to noisy ward atmosphere. Seems to feel strongly about his failure in his relationship with his wife. Stayed up late. **TNS**

Fig. 6.8   (continued)

Nursing interventions (from care plan)	Progress notes
2.6.86 Weekly reassessment.	Colin is feeling worse this week. He complains of headaches and felt as if he had 'flu. Said he had a bad time with his wife yesterday. Gave her 'an earful'. Says she humiliated him in public and is convinced she is part of a business deal to try and get rid of him. Feels he has been used. Seems to have extended his psychotic ideas to include immediate surroundings, e.g. nearby pub and nurses' home. They have been brought into the business deal and are being rented to the hospital. Thinks nurses may be involved in the deal to exclude him from the business venture. Said he will see his wife with the doctor next week and 'thrash out the subject of whether she really wants to leave' then. **D Shields**

References

Altschul A   1972   *Patient–Nurse Interaction. A Study of Interactive Patterns in Acute Psychiatric Wards*. Churchill Livingstone, Edinburgh.

Altschul A   1984   Does good practice need good principles? *Nursing Times*, **80**, 28 & 29.

Coopersmith S   1967   *The Antecedents of Self-esteem*. WH Freeman & Co, San Francisco.

Dietrich G   1978   Teaching psychiatric nursing in the classroom. *Journal of Advanced Nursing*, **3**: 525–534.

Driever MJ   1976   Problem of low self-esteem. In *Introduction to Nursing: An Adaptation Model*, C Roy (Ed). Prentice-Hall, Englewood Cliffs, New Jersey.

Freud S   1911   Psychoanalytical notes upon an autobiographical account of a case of paranoia. In *Three Case Histories*. Collier Books, New York.

Galbreath JG   1980   Sister Callister Roy. In *Nursing Theories* (Nursing Theories Conference Group). Prentice-Hall, Englewood Cliffs, New Jersey.

Jourard SM   1974   *Healthy Personality*. MacMillan, London.

King IM   1971   *Toward a Theory for Nursing*. John Wiley & Sons, New York.

Klein M   1964   *Love, Hate and Reparation*. WW Norton, New York.

Kolb LC   1977   *Modern Clinical Psychiatry*, 9th Ed. WB Saunders, Philadelphia.

Lemert EM   1951   *Social Pathology*. McGraw Hill, New York; Toronto; London.

Levine ME   1969   *Introduction to Clinical Nursing*. FA Davis Co, Philadelphia.

McFarlane EA   1980   Nursing theory: The comparison of four theoretical proposals. *Journal of Advanced Nursing*, **5**: 3–18.

Meize-Grochowski R   1984   An analysis of the concept of trust. *Journal of Advanced Nursing*, **9**: 563–572.

Post F   1982   Paranoid disorders. In *Handbook of Psychiatry 3 – Psychoses of Uncertain Aetiology*. JK Wing & L Wing (Eds). Cambridge University Press.

Riehl JP & Roy C (Eds)   1980   *Conceptual Models for Nursing Practice*. Appleton-Century-Crofts, New York.

Roy C   1976   *Introduction to Nursing: An Adaptation Model*. Prentice-Hall, Englewood Cliffs, New Jersey.

Stuart GW & Sundeen SJ   1983   *Principles and Practice of Psychiatric Nursing*, 2nd Ed. CV Mosby Co, St Louis.

Sullivan HS   1953   *The Interpersonal Theory of Psychiatry*. WW Norton, New York.

Tousley MM   1984   The paranoid fortress of David J. *Journal of Psychosocial Nursing*, **22**, 2.

Towell D   1975   *Understanding Psychiatric Nursing*. Royal College of Nursing, London.

Weddell D   1968   Change in approach. *Psychosocial Nursing*, E Barnes (Ed). Tavistock Publications, London.

Yura H & Walsh MB   1982   *Human Needs and the Nursing Process 2*. Appleton-Century-Crofts, New York.

7

Care plan for an obsessional person, using a cognitive-behavioural model

Verina Wilde

This chapter explains how several models appropriate to therapeutic nursing intervention are integrated in the care of a man with an obsessional disorder.

An *eclectic* approach would require that the most appropriate elements from different models are selected and applied. However, by *integrating* different models, this chapter shows how a thorough understanding of different models (including their limitations) enables the nurse therapist to bring this understanding to bear on the current situation.

Obsessive-compulsive disorders

Samuel Johnson, John Bunyan and Charles Darwin each suffered from an obsessional disorder. Some of their obsessional tendencies could be harnessed usefully, such as collecting, systematically ordering, and organising. Some, however, caused a high degree of discomfort, such as struggling with unacceptable thoughts. The most famous contemporary sufferer was the multimillionaire Howard Hughes, who is reported to have had a strong obsessional fear of contamination.

Excellent reviews of the disorder have been written by Rachman and Hodgson (1980) and Foa and Tillmans (1980). Briefly, an obsessive compulsive disorder is characterised by a recurrent or persistent thought, image, impulse, or action, that is accompanied by a sense of subjective compulsion, and a desire to resist it. An obsession can be described as an intrusive, repetitive thought, image or impulse, that is unacceptable or unwanted, and gives rise to subjective resistance. It generally produces distress and is difficult to control. A compulsion is a repetitive, stereotyped act, that is regarded as excessive by the person performing it. The two major types of compulsive activities or rituals identified by Rachman and Hodgson are cleaning and checking. A third, less common condition, of primary obsessional slowness has been identified by Rachman (1974), Bennun (1980) and Clarke *et al.* (1982).

The incidence of obsessive-compulsive neurosis is quoted as 3% of all neurotic disorders (Black, 1974). My experience as a behavioural nurse therapist is in keeping with this, in that approximately 4% of the people referred to me had a psychiatric diagnosis of obsessive-compulsive neurosis. A much larger group of people presented with complaints of anxiety and depression, and had associated obsessional or compulsive traits. Sometimes these traits were identified by the referrer, but often it was in the course of my behavioural analysis that activities such as checking and ruminating were labelled for the first time. This much larger group of clients, experiencing repetitive, worrying thoughts, and/or being overconcerned with tidiness or the need to check, can be helped enormously by being taught the cognitive and behavioural skills that have been shown to be effective for the less common but more seriously impaired people suffering from obsessive-compulsive neurosis.

I have purposely chosen to describe the application of a cognitive-behavioural model to a client presenting with anxiety symptoms and obsessional traits since he represents the large group of people for whom the model is applicable.

Excellent reviews of the research into the natural history of obsessions and compulsions are available (Black, 1974; Rachman and Hodgson, 1980). To summarise, the disorder is distributed equally amongst men and women, although women are more readily admitted as inpatients. The mean age of onset is the early 20s. There is no evidence that obsessionality is genetically determined. However, there appears to be distinctive parent behaviour in the families of obsessional people. Rachman (1976) suggested that both cleaners and checkers experienced excessive parental control. He observed that while parents of cleaners appeared to be over-controlling and protective, the parents of checkers appeared over-controlling and over-critical. These processes appear to play an important part in generating and maintaining behaviour tendencies such as timidity and over-dependence, and these dispositions provide fertile soil for the growth of obsessions and compulsions.

There is evidence to suggest that people suffering from the disorder are more intelligent than average (see studies quoted in Black, 1974 and Rachman and Hodgson, 1980). Black suggests that intelligent people are more capable of abstract thinking which predisposes them to ruminations.

There are higher rates of celibacy in people with obsessive-compulsive disorders and a frequent occurrence of sexual and marital difficulties.

Rachman and Hodgson (1980) found that most cleaners reported a sudden onset of the disorder, whilst most checkers reported a gradual onset.

The relationship between obsessionality and depression is complex. In some instances, improvement in depression is accompanied by a reduction in obsession, while Paykel et al. (1976) found that recovery from depression left the average level of obsessional traits unaffected. Capstick (1975) reported on the value of antidepressant medication in overcoming obsessional problems. Rachman and Hodgson (1980) conclude that there is some evidence to suggest that obsessions can promote the maintenance of depression. In a small number of cases (the incidence varies between 0 and 3%) an obsessional condition can change into a psychotic one, but there is no close relationship between obsessive-compulsive disorders and schizophrenia.

Rachman and Hodgson (1980) classify the disorder into five categories: checking, washing/cleaning, slowness/repetition, doubting/conscientious and ruminating. There is some evidence (Sher et al., 1983) that checkers are deficient in their memory for actions which may account for their need to check to reassure their 'did I or didn't I?' doubt.

Choosing an appropriate model

The person presented in this chapter was treated using a cognitive-behavioural model and its theoretical bases have been well documented (Bandura, 1969; Rimm and Masters, 1979; Foa and Tillmans, 1980). Briefly, the features that distinguish cognitive-behavioural methods from other treatments are that they are concerned more with factors that maintain symptoms and abnormal behaviours than with original causes, they are based on psychological experimentation, and they are designed to encourage self help (Gelder, 1986).

With regard to the treatment of obsessive compulsive disorders Turner et al. (1979) pointed out that prior to the late 1960s when behaviourally orientated treatment strategies were developed for the problem, obsessive-compulsive disorders were notoriously resistant to treatment no matter what the theoretical persuasion of the therapist. Cawley (1974) described the psychodynamic approach to obsessional disorders but concluded that it was difficult to assess the efficacy of treatment.

Foa and Tillmans (1980) reviewed the experimental evidence for the effectiveness of various behavioural interventions with obsessive-compulsive disorders, including desensitisation in real life, aversion relief conditioning, flooding and response prevention, and participant modelling, real-life exposure and response prevention. Foa and Tillmans (1980) and Rachman and Hodgson (1980) described the various behavioural formulations of obsessive-compulsive neurosis including Mowrer's avoidance conditioning model and Teasdales avoidance/avoidance conflict. Foa and Tillmans concluded that a combination of exposure and response prevention (first used by Meyer in 1966) appeared to be the treatment of choice for ritualistic behaviour.

With regard to the treatment of obsessional thoughts, research has centred on the two techniques of thought stopping and satiation. Thought stopping was first described by Wolpe in 1958 although Tryon (1979) pointed out that similar procedures have been in use for over a century. The technique consists of teaching the client to interrupt his thoughts, at first by a sudden external distraction and later by mental distraction. Lombardo and Turner (1979) and Martin (1982) described the effective use of thought stopping in individual case studies. A controlled study reported by Stern (1978) failed to demonstrate the effectiveness of thought stopping, while Arrick *et al.* (1981) demonstrated that thought stopping alone, covert assertion alone, or a combination of these treatments, were both more effective than a control procedure. Kirk (1983) found thought stopping a useful procedure used in clinical practice.

The more recently developed technique of satiation involves the client being encouraged to produce the thoughts on request, and to hold on to them, rather than curtailing the ruminations (Rachman, 1976). Parkinson and Rachman (1980) showed that brief repeated exposure to the thoughts, with relaxation exercises, was more effective than prolonged exposure to the intrusive thoughts. This form of habituation has similarities with thought stopping. Emmelkamp and Kwee (1977) compared the effects of thought stopping and prolonged exposure in imagination and found that both techniques could be effective.

To sum up, it is possible that the effect brought about by thought stopping and satiation is the result of one and the same process. Although the techniques differ with regard to the continuity of exposure, exposure to the worrying thoughts is common to both techniques and the effect of both techniques is likely to be based on habituation.

Much research has been carried out to test the effectiveness of training nurses to use a behavioural model of care. A three year research project was started at the Maudsley Hospital in 1972 with the aim of producing nurses with a broad range of behavioural theory and practice who could work autonomously. This culminated in the establishment of a nationally recognised course of 18 months duration by the then Joint Board of Clinical Nursing Studies (now the English National Board). The research project showed that the nurse therapists were at least as effective as psychiatrists and psychologists (Marks *et al.*, 1975, 1977). Some people were not impressed at the time, and an analogy was made that teaching nurses to be behavioural psychotherapists was like teaching lorry drivers to fly aeroplanes!

Marks *et al.* (1978) reported that obsessive-compulsive clients treated by nurse therapists improved significantly in time spent on rituals per day, discomfort during rituals, total obsessive behaviour, and work adjustment. Their pilot study showed nurse therapists to deliver cost-effective treatment, and led to a more detailed study of Marks and Waters (1984) into the cost-effectiveness of nurse therapists working in primary health care.

Bird *et al.* (1979) reviewed the developments, controversies and implications of nurse therapists in psychiatry. Lindley *et al.* (1984) reported on a national follow-up of nurse therapists trained on the ENB course 650. The majority worked as autonomous clinical nurse therapists and were widely accepted by nursing and other colleagues. Lindley *et al.* concluded that more training centres were needed.

A number of case studies of obsessive-compulsive clients have been published where therapy has been successfully carried out by nurse therapists (Keen, 1982; Farrington, 1983; Mercer, 1984).

Nurse Therapy has been built on a solid foundation of evaluative research in the relatively short time span of a decade.

(Brooker, 1984: p.3)

In summary, there is much evidence to support the use of behavioural psychotherapy for obsessional-compulsive disorders and the effectiveness of nurses as behavioural psychotherapists. Nurse therapists work as autonomous therapists, responsible for the behavioural assessment, definition of problems, evaluation of progress, problem orientated record keeping and appreciation of research methods.

Outline and critique of the cognitive-behavioural model

Comprehensive reviews of the origins and development of behaviour therapy and cognitive therapy are available elsewhere (Rimm and Masters, 1979; Yates, 1970; Lazarus, 1971; Agras *et al.*, 1979; Barker and Fraser, 1985). Here I propose to restrict the discussion to the principles of present day behavioural psychotherapy and then to give an outline of the cognitive-behavioural model of care.

The following is a summary of the principles of behavioural psychotherapy. Behavioural assessment and treatment concentrate more on the behaviour itself than on a presumed underlying cause. The assumption is that abnormal behaviour is acquired and maintained in the same way that normal behaviour is learned, and that it can be treated through the application of behavioural principles. Many types of abnormal behaviour, formerly regarded as illnesses in themselves or as signs and symptoms of illness, are better construed as problems of social adaptation. Treatment involves analysis of the problem into its component parts, and setting specific goals or targets in relation to these. The therapist adapts her method of treatment to the individual client's problems. Behaviour therapy is organised around an explicit testable conceptual framework, and the techniques used can be described with sufficient precision to be measured objectively and to be replicated. Innovative research strategies allow rigorous evaluation of specific methods applied to particular problems.

Contemporary behaviour therapy draws from a wide range of theoretical concepts, including Pavlov's classical conditioning, and Thorndike and Skinner's instrumental or operant conditioning.

Mowrer linked these two forms of conditioning together with his two factor theory when he asserted in 1947 that a fear response acquired by classical conditioning was maintained by operant conditioning (see Barker and Fraser, 1985). Bandura (1969) advocated a social learning theory, since he believed that behaviour was learned vicariously rather than by direct experience. He showed that imitation or modelling techniques could be used for a wide range of problems.

More recently, several psychologists and psychotherapists have developed specific therapeutic techniques directed at the mental processes that accompany problem behaviour. Mahoney (1974) developed the concept of cognitive restructuring, and Meichenbaum (1977) the concept of self-instructional training or coping self-talk. Ellis (1962) developed a type of psychotherapy which he termed Rational Emotive Therapy, and Beck (1976) introduced his concept of cognitive therapy. These four therapists viewed the individual's disturbed patterns of behaviour as a function of certain thinking errors, which are in turn a result of a dysfunctional belief system. Beck's approach helps the patient learn about the relationship between his patterns of thinking, his emotions and his behaviour, and then helps him change his thinking patterns, and thus change his emotional and behavioural responses.

There are differing views as to the range of problems that are suitable for a behavioural approach. Marks *et al.* (1977) viewed behavioural methods as forming the treatment of choice for only 10% of all adult psychiatric outpatients. Barker and Fraser (1985) on the other hand have investigated the possibilities of a more radical behavioural model where all patients are viewed as people with problems of social adaptation or psychological instability, and where a wide range of problems of living are amenable to remediation via an extensive repertoire of behaviour change procedures.

I support Barker and Wilson's (1985) view of contemporary behaviour therapy as a broadly based therapeutic system which reflects the subtle interplay between the person, and his biophysical, social, political and economic worlds.

At the heart of the cognitive-behavioural model

of care is the concept of the behavioural analysis, as the basis of assessment. Kanfer and Saslow (1965) provided a useful outline for the analysis, which is summarised below.

(a) *Analysis of the problem situation.* The person's major complaints are categorised into classes of behavioural excesses and deficits. For each excess or deficit, the frequency, intensity, duration and stimulus conditions are described. The client's behavioural assets are also listed, for utilisation in the behavioural programme.

(b) *Clarification of the problem situation.* The people and circumstances that maintain the problem behaviour are considered, and the consequences of these behaviours to the client and others in his environment are identified.

(c) *Motivational analysis.* A hierarchy of reinforcing people, events and objects are established to permit utilisation of appropriate reinforcing behaviour by the therapist and significant others.

(d) *Development analysis.* Questions are asked about the person's physical state, his sociocultural experience and his characteristic behavioural development.

(e) *Analysis of self-control.* The person's methods and degree of self-control are examined. Persons or events that have successfully reinforced self-controlling behaviours are considered.

(f) *Analysis of social relationships.* The individual's social network is examined to evaluate the significance of people in the person's environment who have some influence over the problematic behaviours, or who in turn are influenced by the patient for his own satisfactions. These interpersonal relationships are reviewed in order to plan the potential participation of significant others in the treatment programme. The review also helps the therapist to consider the range of actual social relationships in which the patient needs to function.

(g) *Analysis of the social-cultural-physical environment.* Here the preceding analysis of the person's behaviour as an individual is extended to include a consideration of the norms of his usual environment. Agreements and discrepancies between the person's idiosyncratic life patterns and the norms of his environment are defined so that the importance of these factors can be decided when formulating treatment goals.

Lazarus (1973, 1985) provides another excellent structure for assessment and therapy, which he has termed multimodal therapy. A fundamental premise of this approach is that clients are troubled by a multitude of specific problems that may require a wide range of specific treatments. Assessment and treatment are organised across seven modalities: behaviour, affect, sensation, imagery, cognition, interpersonal relationships and biological factors. BASIC IB is an acronym derived from this sequence, but for convenience as an *aide-mémoire*, Lazarus uses D (for drugs) to stand for the biological modality, resulting in the more compelling acronym BASIC ID, or BASIC I.D. (I.D. as in identity).

The model used in the case presented in this chapter is based on Lazarus' multimodal therapy, but includes factors from the Kanfer and Saslow (1965) approach, since Lazarus' BASIC ID model does not address factors such as political, and socio-cultural events. The case illustrates how a detailed behavioural analysis can identify a number of additional problems not identified by a medical diagnosis. Each of these problems can be tackled with specific interventions which may not have otherwise appeared relevant to the presenting problem. For example it may emerge that a person referred with obsessional tendencies experiences difficulties in the interpersonal skills modality and requires social skills and assertion training in addition to the more obvious exposure and response prevention techniques. Turner *et al.* (1979) also found that individuals with obsessive-compulsive disorders frequently present with additional symptoms, and they suggested the use of specific strategies to deal with related and unrelated symptoms such as depression, marital problems and social skills deficits.

With regard to the effectiveness of the behavioural model in the treatment of obsessional problems, Foa (1979) suggested that severely depressed people and those who believe their fears are realistic may fail to respond to exposure and response prevention. Salkovskis and Warwick (1985) successfully treated an obsessional client with over-valued ideation and depression using a combination of Beck's cognitive therapy and exposure.

From personal experience and discussion with other behaviour therapists, there appear to be certain clients whose obsessive-compulsive behaviour seems to have a strong positive function for the client, such as avoidance of sex, or over-reliance on the spouse, but the client declines offers of help for these associated problems. A shortcoming in the behavioural approach is that the feelings engendered in the therapist when the client is not succeeding, are not accommodated. Resistant clients, or clients who do not do what the therapist asks them to, can cause the therapist to doubt his or her effectiveness, and it can be a relief when such a client drops out of therapy. The dynamic psychotherapy view of transference and counter-transference may be of some use to the therapist in these cases (although other behaviour therapists may not agree with me!). Paradoxical Intention (Frankl, 1960) and Strategic Family Therapy (Cade, 1980; Simon and Axford, 1983) can be useful when working with resistance in the client or the family. Wilde *et al.* (1985) describe a course where nurses were trained to use Strategic Family Therapy.

The refreshing feature of Lazarus' multimodal therapy is that although most techniques used are drawn from cognitive-behaviour therapy, practitioners select methods that are demonstrably effective, and while this points in most cases to cognitive-behavioural procedures, the multimodal framework facilitates the use of methods from family systems, communications, training, Gestalt therapy, psychodrama, and many other orientations when the situation demands.

Before moving on to the actual history it may be helpful to look at Fig. 7.1 which is a flow chart of the cognitive-behavioural model.

Client history

Colin was twenty-two, and lived with his parents and brother. He worked as a mechanic in a local garage and his spare time was spent watching a variety of sports and umpiring football matches. He enjoyed going out to quiet pubs with a friend, but felt shy of meeting new people and had never had a regular girlfriend.

Over a period of a few months he began to feel tense and panicky in situations he normally coped with. His symptoms became so intense he consulted his GP, who prescribed chlordiazepoxide tablets. Colin disliked the drowsy effect of the tranquillisers and returned to his GP. By this time his symptoms had worsened and he was taking time off work. He had become preoccupied with worries about political instability in various parts of the world, and ruminated on the possibility of nuclear war breaking out.

His GP referred him to a psychiatrist who described Colin as having symptoms of an anxiety state. He identified Colin's obsessional traits but considered these to be only mildly incapacitating, and he excluded clinical depression from his diagnosis. He prescribed lorazepam tablets, but appreciated Colin's apprehension about taking tranquillisers. He referred Colin to me as he thought Colin would benefit from a behavioural approach to his anxiety.

Assessment

The behavioural interview has a structure which acts as a framework on which the interviewer hangs questions. The basic structure (in this case, the BASIC ID) influences the outcome of the interview but the framework is flexible. It provides the interviewer with some guidance as to the topics that might usefully be covered but it does not dictate the actual questions to be asked. It was important to have a plan of the broad areas I wanted to cover in the interview without having the session too highly structured, with a list of questions to ask. This latter style might have led to me fitting Colin's problems to my questions.

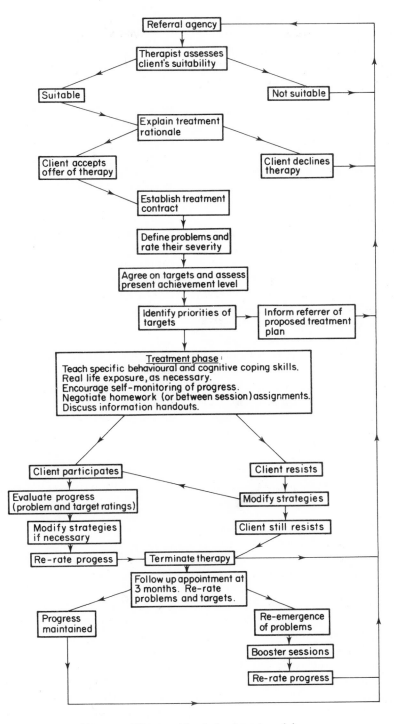

Fig. 7.1   The cognitive-behavioural model

Colin was very flustered at the beginning of the interview, blushing noticeably and stumbling over his words. I explained simply what the plan of the session was, and asked what had led up to him coming to see me. This gave Colin the opportunity to describe the most significant events or problems from his point of view. My questions at the beginning of the interview were lower-order questions, which were simple, involving recall of information. As Colin relaxed I moved on to higher-order questions which required him to analyse situations, make predictions, and discuss complex ideas. Examples of higher-order questions are, 'What would happen if you did that?', or 'What would be so bad about that?'.

Figure 7.2 includes a summary of the behavioural analysis, and the second column contains a breakdown of Colin's presenting behaviour and cognitions.

We agreed to meet in a week's time, and before he left I gave him a copy of the Life History Questionnaire (Lazarus, 1971). I asked him to complete it for next time, when we would look over it together. Care must be taken when asking people to fill in questionnaires and record sheets that they are within their intellectual and educational capabilities, to ensure a feeling of competence in the client. Colin was relieved when I reassured him that a lot of people worried about their spelling or grammar being correct, but that it was the information and not the presentation that was important.

Colin returned to the second session with the questionnaire impeccably filled in. We completed the assessment during this session. The other assessment tools used were the Fear Questionnaire, the Areas of Impairment Rating Scale, the Anxiety Rating Scale, and the Beck Depression Inventory.

The Fear Questionnaire (Marks and Mathews, 1979) can show how widespread the person's anxieties are. A number of situations are listed and the person is provided with a nine point scale. Colin was asked to choose a number from nought to eight, from the scale, to indicate how likely he would be to avoid a situation. He was then asked to rate on a similar scale how troublesome he found various feelings, such as feeling irritable, angry, depressed, or being troubled by worrying thoughts.

The Areas of Impairment Rating Scale uses the same nine point scale (often referred to as a 'nought-to-eight scale') to rate the degree of impairment that the problems cause to the person's work, home management, social leisure activities, private leisure activities and family relationships.

The Anxiety Rating Scale has five questions, relating to the frequency, duration, and intensity of anxious feelings experienced by the client, who again is asked to use a nought-to-eight scale for each question. An example question is:

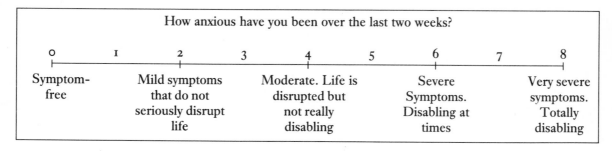

The client is asked to circle the number which most closely describes their symptoms.

The Beck Depression Inventory (Beck *et al.*, 1980) is viewed by many as the best available measure of the severity of depression (Barker, 1985). It can be used as a screening assessment to see if any depression exists. I used it with Colin as he had described feeling depressed at times, and had reported having lost interest in previously enjoyable activities. Beck has published norms which allow us to judge how severely depressed a client is. The scale covers 21 aspects of affective disorder, including feelings of shame, guilt, sadness, eating, sleeping, sex, decision making, work

Fig. 7.2 Behavioural analysis and treatment using Lazarus' multimodal BASIC ID

Modality	Problem/present behaviour	Target	Strategy
Behaviour:	Has to listen to news every half-hour on radio or TV.	To listen to news once a day only.	Coping self-talk and response prevention. Diary of urges and responses.
(a) Excesses	Returns to car to check ignition is switched off, and door locked.	To resist checking car ignition and door.	
	Checks jobs at work over meticulously.	To resist checking jobs at work.	
	Possessions kept in very orderly fashion.	To tolerate untidiness and disorder.	Exposure and response prevention.
	Increased alcohol consumption since anxiety problem.	To return to previous level of consumption.	Self-monitoring, daily allowance and self-talk.
	Increased appetite and weight gain (eats when anxious)	To regain control of dietary intake, and lose 10 lb.	Monitor intake, set daily allowance, increase exercise.
	Worried that he blushes easily.	To reduce the 'awfulness' of this (decatastrophising).	Cognitive restructing: 'so what, if I'm blushing, it will pass'.
	Loses temper at least once a day.	To put his point of view across without losing temper.	Assertive skills training.
	Leaves shops because tense.	To go into large shops and stay as long as he wishes.	Graded target setting and coping self-talk.
(b) Deficits	Unable to relax. Unable to sit still.	To recognise early signals of tension and to prevent escalation.	Relaxation exercises.
	Poor eye contact.	To be able to look at people during conversations.	Role play, and homework assignments.
	Lack of assertive skills, e.g. finds it very difficult to give his point of view; finds it difficult to disagree with friends and workmates.	To be able to put into words his ideas and thoughts. To value his own opinion. To be able to voice his disagreement where appropriate.	Cognitive restructuring 'My opinion is important'. Assertive skills training.
(c) Assets	Has one good friend he can confide in.	To increase social contacts.	Diary of social contacts.
	Has maintained his job, and social activities despite feeling very anxious.	To continue to attend work and social activities.	Anxiety management training.

Fig. 7.2   (continued)

Modality	Problem/present behaviour	Target	Strategy
Affect	Feels anxious most of the time. Has 2–3 bad panic attacks a day.	To learn to control panicky feelings.	Distraction techniques, coping self-talk, cognitive restructuring.
	Depressed at times. Has lost interest in previously pleasurable activities.	To recognise assets. To control worrying thoughts. To increase frequency of enjoyable pastimes.	Cognitive restructuring. Diary of activities.
	Gets anxious eating in public.	To have a pub lunch once a week with a friend.	Planned exposure and coping self-talk.
Sensations	'Butterflies' in stomach. Breathless. Feels sick. Tense muscles, especially thighs. Feels hot.	To reduce the frequency of these sensations. To understand why they occur. To use them as signals to start anxiety management techniques.	Education about the physiological nature of anxiety. Information booklet (anxiety). Relaxation exercises. Controlled breathing. Coping self-talk.
Imagery	Nightmares in the past.	To reduce the unpleasantness of the nightmares.	Relaxation exercises at bedtime Rehearsal relief of nightmare. (I described the strategy that we could use, but the nightmares stopped before we put it into practice.)
Cognitions	'I'm going to be sick.' Worries about world events, political instability and possible nuclear war. 'Have I switched the car engine off? I must go back and check.' 'People think I'm thick.' 'I look a fool.' 'I can't stop eating, I'll be as fat as a pig.'	To recognise negative, worrying or self-defeating thoughts, and restructure them in a more positive way. To be able to interrupt repetitive thoughts. To increase self-esteem	Diary of frequency of worrying thoughts. Cognitive restructuring. Encourage participation in pressure groups. Thought stopping.
	'I don't want to be a mechanic for the rest of my life.' Worries about Dad dying, although he is in good health.	To explore other career options.	Career opportunities – public library index. Consult Job Centre. Educational Advisory Service.
	Worries about learning new refereeing rules.	To know and understand refereeing rules	Graded homework assignments.

Fig. 7.2 (continued)

Modality	Problem/present behaviour	Target	Strategy
Interpersonal	Feels parents have over-protected him. Good circle of acquaintances. One good friend. Easily embarrassed. Feels self-conscious and tongue-tied with girls. Has difficulty dealing with teasing from workmates. Has difficulty in giving his opinion.	To feel more confidence in conversations, especially with girls. To speak more slowly and clearly. To 'give as good as I get'. To see opinion as important.	Social skills training. Role play, homework assignments. Coping self-talk. Cognitive restructuring.
Drugs	Chlordiazepoxide (discontinued – made him drowsy) Lorazepam 1 mg PRN.	To manage anxiety symptoms with self-coping strategies. To discontinue anxiolytic medication.	Positive coping self-talk. Relaxation exercises. Breathing exercises. Planned reduction of PRN medication.

and physical appearance. Each item has four statements and the client is asked to select the statement which most closely represents how they feel. Table 7.1 shows the interpretation of scores on the Beck Depression Inventory (Burns, 1980).

Table 7.1 Interpretation of scores on the Beck Depression Inventory (Burns, 1980)

1–10	These ups and downs considered normal.
11–16	Mild mood disturbance.
17–20	Borderline clinical depression.
21–30	Moderate depression.
31–40	Severe depression.
Over 40	Extreme depression.

Colin's pretreatment score was 17, which was within the borderline clinical depression category. As a result, I decided to keep a check on his mood, and to observe for depressed thinking styles as therapy progressed.

The last part of Colin's pretreatment assessment consisted of asking him to keep a record of urges to check his car ignition. He was given a homework record sheet, and asked to indicate on this each

time he resisted the urge, and each time he gave in and checked. He was also asked to write down any upsetting thoughts he had as soon as they occurred, and to indicate how long they had lasted. This self-recording of worrying thoughts would give me a clearer idea of the content of the thoughts, and would show Colin that although it felt as if he was constantly troubled by the thoughts, that there were in fact periods when he was free of them.

To summarise, Colin's assessment involved the following.

1 Face-to-face interviews where information was obtained by direct questioning and observation of non-verbal behaviour.

2 Self-assessment questionnaires (the Fear Questionnaire, Areas of Impairment Questionnaire, Life History Questionnaire and Anxiety Questionnaire and the Beck Depression Inventory).

3 Self-monitoring of the frequency of problem behaviour and cognitions.

It was explained to Colin that we would be able to repeat the self-assessment ratings at various stages in therapy to monitor his progress. Colin's pretreatment scores can be seen in Figs 7.7–7.9.

Problems and goals

Following the assessment, Colin was asked to select the problems that were of most concern to him, and to rate their severity on two nought-to-eight scales (Fig. 7.3).

Scale 1   *Behaviour*
This problem interferes with my normal activities:

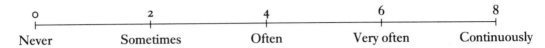

0	2	4	6	8
Never	Sometimes	Often	Very often	Continuously

Scale 2   *Emotions*
This problem upsets me:

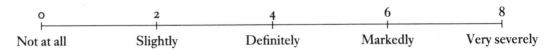

0	2	4	6	8
Not at all	Slightly	Definitely	Markedly	Very severely

For each of these problems, a target was drawn up, and these were also rated on two scales, the first measuring success in achieving the target, and the second rating the degree of difficulty with regard to that target (Fig. 7.4).

Scale 1   *Behaviour*

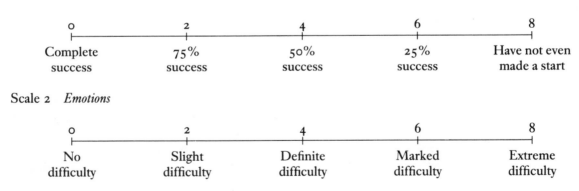

0	2	4	6	8
Complete success	75% success	50% success	25% success	Have not even made a start

Scale 2   *Emotions*

0	2	4	6	8
No difficulty	Slight difficulty	Definite difficulty	Marked difficulty	Extreme difficulty

The problem and targets were both rated on two scales because improvement in behaviour and emotions is often out of synchrony. Changes in behaviour generally precede changes in anxiety levels, and it is necessary to monitor both aspects separately. It is important to select a problem from the list that can be tackled most easily. This is more likely to ensure early success for the client, and increase his motivation to tackle more complex problems. Targets need to be realistic and achievable, and often need to be broken down into a series of small steps of increasing difficulty. The wording of the problem and targets should be in the client's style of language, whilst being stated in precise and measurable terms.

Intervention

The strategies used in therapy with Colin and the coping skills taught to him are summarised in the fourth column of Fig. 7.2. Here, I will select the

Fig. 7.3   Assessment of problem severity

	Problem	Scale 1	Scale 2
A	Upsetting thoughts come into mind (e.g., nuclear war starting) that I can't shift.	6	7
B	I get tense and panicky and I can't relax.	7	8
C	I have to go back and check that I have done things, for instance, that I have switched the car engine off.	6	7
D	I am concerned about things being tidy and in their right place.	2	7
E	I get anxious eating in front of other people.	7	7
F	I get anxious in crowds and I avoid busy shops.	7	7
G	I find it difficult to say what I mean, and to put my point of view across to other people.	7	8

Fig. 7.4   Assessment of degree of success and difficulty in achieving targets

	Targets	Scale 1	Scale 2
A	To control negative worrying thoughts, and to restructure them in a more positive way.	8	7
B	To be able to relax and control my panicky feelings.	7	7
C	To resist the urge to go back and check the car ignition.	8	7
D	To resist the urge to put everything back in their right places.	8	8
E	To have a pub lunch with a friend once a week.	7	8
F	To browse around busy shops and to be able to queue at the check-out counter.	6	7
G	To say what I am thinking, without losing my temper.	8	8

most important elements of the intervention to use as illustrations.

The first thing we tackled was Colin's anxiety about learning some new sports rules. He had found that his anxiety about being able to apply the new refereeing rules (due to lack of assertion) was interfering with his ability to concentrate on learning them. We broke down the task into a number of steps, and allocated a step a night as homework. Colin was asked to keep a homework diary of his progress throughout the week. When we reviewed his homework (Fig. 7.5) he was pleased to report that he had been able to concentrate on the task for an average of 45 minutes each day, and that his difficulty in concentrating (rated on a nought-to-eight scale) had decreased, and his satisfaction on completion

of the task (also rated on a nought-to-eight scale) had increased, as the week progressed.

The next problem was Colin's urge to check his car ignition: self-monitoring having revealed that he had been tempted to check 43 times in a week, and had been unable to resist each time. He stated that he only felt the urge to check when he was on his own, so real-life exposure and response prevention in my presence were inappropriate. Instead, we discussed the principles of response prevention, and various strategies that he could implement to resist the urge. These focused mainly on positive coping statements. I guided him through an imaginary scene, where he experienced a strong urge to check the car but used positive coping self-talk and distraction techniques to resist.

I asked Colin to keep a diary of urges to check,

Fig. 7.5   Homework diary

Date	Daily task	Time spent	Concentration difficulty 0–8	Pleasure on completion 0–8	Comments
25th April	Read through half the rules.	40 mins.	7	0	Found it very difficult.
25th April	Read through second half of rules.	45 mins.	7	2	
27th April	5–6 rules each night for the rest of the week.	45 mins.	6	3	Read laws in the morning.
28th April	After reading the rules, close the book and write down what you can remember, then check this with the rule book.	30 mins.	7	1	Read in the morning.
29th April		1 hour.	7	2	Half-hour in morning, half-hour in evening
30th April		45 mins.	6	4	Surprised I was able to remember some.
1st May		30 mins.	5	4	
2nd May		45 mins.	3	5	

and we reviewed this each week. Colin found that he was most tempted to go back to the car when he had gone indoors for the last time at night. I asked him to come up with some ideas to help him resist going outside to check. He suggested making a small sign to place near the door in the porch, with the initials D.B.D. (Don't Be Daft!). This served as a very useful reminder to stop if he got as far as the porch on his way back to check, and was probably more effective because it was his own suggestion.

In four weeks he had reduced his checking behaviour to zero and was rarely troubled by urges to check (see Fig. 7.12).

Having been successful with this problem we moved on to tackle Colin's intrusive thoughts. He kept a record of these diligently and it was apparent that they fell into two categories, self-esteem and world events.

In the area of self-esteem we identified a number of thinking errors, or 'cognitive distortions' (Beck, 1980). Colin often displayed all-or-nothing thinking, for example, 'I am not a total success, therefore I am a complete failure'. He tended to exaggerate

mishaps, and to catastrophise, imagining dreadful consequences of his behaviour. He tended to discount positive aspects of a situation and was much more willing to identify his weaknesses than his strengths. He often jumped to conclusions about himself without much evidence. For example, he told me that people always laughed at him when he gave his point of view, but on reflection admitted that there was only one person, a workmate, who occasionally made fun of his views.

Colin was taught to identify thinking errors, and to practise answering the automatic thoughts with more accurate, positive statements. An example of his cognitive restructuring homework is given in Fig. 7.6.

Colin was very distressed by repetitive thoughts of political instability, threats of war, and nuclear accidents. They could occur spontaneously but more usually occurred whilst listening to the news, or waiting for the news to come on the television or radio. I thought carefully about how best to help Colin with these thoughts since to a certain extent they were reasonable fears but had escalated to unmanageable proportions. We agreed that the fact

Fig. 7.6 Positive restructuring homework

Negative thought	More positive answer
Everything is an effort. The harder I try to do things the less I do.	Any little thing I do (like clean my football boots) I'll give myself praise.
I hate myself for exaggerating the truth when talking to a lad in the pub.	At least I'm doing it less than I used to.
Dad is late coming home from work. I panic about all the things that could have happened to him.	He'll just be working late. Do something to take your mind off worrying.
Why has Bill (workmate) kept running to the radio and shaking his head? I'll have to ask him, maybe there is a world crisis.	He has been listening to a report about gas bills.

that he felt so powerless was contributing to the high level of anxiety, causing him to ruminate on the thoughts. We agreed that it would be sensible to try to gain some control on the ruminations, so that his concern could be channelled more effectively. A combination of thought stopping and cognitive restructuring was used with the 'world events' anxieties and I mentioned that some people channelled their concerns into activity and political pressure. Colin was interested in finding out more about local pressure groups, so I suggested he make enquiries at the library about local branches of the Ecology Party, Friends of the Earth, Greenpeace and the Campaign for Nuclear Disarmament.

This was the real turning point in Colin's treatment. He plucked up courage to join two of the local groups, and as a result, his social contacts widened. He had an excellent opportunity to practise giving his opinion in discussions, and most importantly, he felt he was no longer powerless in the nuclear debate.

A number of our sessions at this point focused on building up Colin's repertoire of social skills. Special attention was paid to improving his eye contact, slowing down his speech and capitalising on his asset of listening.

Colin noticed that he became even more concerned about tidiness around this time, and we initiated a programme to tackle this. He agreed to purposely untidy his bedroom and to move items around into untidy positions each day, while resisting any urges to replace them in their 'proper positions'. He kept a very specific diary sheet of urges and resistance from day to day, and was

pleased to note an 80% ability to resist in the first week and a 100% ability to resist in the second and subsequent weeks. He had thus been able to transfer the skill of response prevention, learned in relation to checking the car ignition, to this area of concern.

I asked Colin to keep a diary of social activities at the beginning, middle and end of therapy, and there was a dramatic increase in the range of social activities that he engaged in, as therapy progressed. He reported that many of his frustrations at work were because he did not enjoy his job, and that he would like to have more contact with people. He had obtained a Careers Directory from the library, and expressed an interest in working with children. He decided to enrol for night classes to study for some more O levels, while remaining in his existing job for the time being. I was relieved at this decision, since it would give him the opportunity to be assertive with his awkward workmate, rather than escaping by changing jobs.

An interesting point to note in Colin's treatment was that while certain behaviours were tackled with specific interventions, the emphasis was on teaching new coping skills which could be applied in a number of different situations. Colin was able to generalise skills learned to new situations. For instance, he tackled his fear of crowds, eating in public and of busy shops, using graded targets and coping self-talk, without any specific intervention by me.

Colin and I had a total of ten sessions, each lasting approximately one hour. Assessment ratings were repeated on the sixth and tenth sessions. We had a follow-up appointment three months after completion of therapy, when the ratings were repeated again.

Evaluation

Colin was really pleased with his progress, but even he was surprised when we compared the results of the rating scales and the frequency counts of problem behaviour taken at the beginning and end of therapy. The Fear Questionnaire, the Areas of Impairment Questionnaire, the Anxiety Questionnaire and the Beck Depression Inventory all showed a marked decrease in scores, and hence improvement (Figs 7.7–7.9).

The problem and target ratings showed a similar improvement (decrease) in scores (Figs 7.10 and 7.11). Scale 1 measured behavioural change and Scale 2 measured emotional change for both problem and target ratings.

As can be seen on the graph (Fig. 7.12) the frequency of actual checking and urges to check had reduced to zero by the ninth week of therapy.

At follow-up, three months after therapy, the ratings were repeated and on every measure Colin had at least maintained his post-treatment scores. On the Fear Questionnaire, the Anxiety Questionnaire and the Beck Depression Inventory, he had made further improvements since termination of therapy. He reported that he had commenced evening classes for Psychology and Sociology O

Fig. 7.7   Fear Questionnaire ratings

Rating	Maximum score	Pre therapy	Mid therapy	Post therapy	3 month follow-up
Main fear (crowded places)	8	7	3	2	1
Avoidance of other situations (listed)	120	62	48	30	25
Anxiety and depression	40	28	13	9	7
Present state of phobic symptoms	8	6	3	2	1

Fig. 7.8   Areas of impairment ratings

Area	Maximum score	Pre therapy	Mid therapy	Post therapy	3 month follow-up
Work	8	6	3	2	1
Home	8	4	2	0	0
Social leisure activities	8	7	5	2	2
Private leisure activities	8	6	2	1	0
Relationship with parents	8	1	0	0	0
Relationship with friends	8	5	3	2	1

Fig. 7.9   Anxiety Questionnaire and Beck Depression Inventory

Rating scale	Maximum score	Pre therapy	Mid therapy	Post therapy	3 month follow-up
Anxiety Questionnaire	40	29	23	5	3
Beck Depression Inventory	63	17	10	3	3

Fig. 7.10 Problem ratings. Scale 1 (behaviour), Scale 2 (how much it upsets Colin): maximum score on each scale is 8

Problems	Scale (1 or 2)	Pre therapy	Mid therapy	Post therapy	3 month follow-up
Recurrent thoughts of nuclear war	1 2	6 7	4 5	3 3	1 2
Tense and panicky, can't relax	1 2	7 8	3 4	2 3	1 1
Checking car ignition	1 2	6 7	1 2	0 1	0 0
Things having to be in 'proper' place	1 2	2 7	3 4	0 0	0 0
Anxious eating in front of others	1 2	7 7	2 2	0 2	0 1
Anxious in crowds and busy shops	1 2	7 7	2 3	0 2	0 0
Difficulty in expressing myself	1 2	7 8	4 6	3 4	2 3

Fig. 7.11 Target ratings. Scale 1 (success), Scale 2 (difficulty): maximum score on each scale is 8

Targets	Scale (1 or 2)	Pre therapy	Mid therapy	Post therapy	3 month follow-up
Control worrying thoughts and restructure positively	1 2	8 7	3 3	1 3	1 2
To relax and control panicky feelings	1 2	7 7	3 3	1 2	1 1
To resist urge to check ignition	1 2	8 7	1 1	0 0	0 0
To resist putting things in proper places	1 2	8 8	5 5	0 0	0 0
To have pub lunch once a week with friend	1 2	7 8	4 6	2 3	0 1
To browse in busy shops and queue at check-out	1 2	6 7	5	2	0 0
To speak mind without losing temper	1 2	8 8	5 6	3 4	2 3

level, and that he was continuing to take part in local pressure group activities. He had recently been to a disco, and had asked a girl for a dance, something that he had never before been able to do. He summed up his view of therapy by saying that he had learned that there were many areas of life that he had previously been dissatisfied with, but that he had previously felt were out of his control. He had realised that he could take control of these areas and that as a result he had a much more positive view of himself and the future.

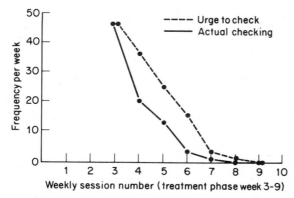

Fig. 7.12 Frequency of urges to check and actual checking of car ignition

Critique of the model in use

A common criticism of behaviour therapy is that it deals with symptoms, rather than the whole person. I hope that it is clear from the discussion that attention was paid to emotional, political, educational, vocational and interactional factors, as well as to presenting symptoms.

An interesting comparison can be made between Colin's psychiatric diagnosis of 'anxiety state' and the behavioural formulation of his problems. As a result of the behavioural analysis, we identified obsessional and compulsive traits, social skills deficits, and assertion difficulties, that were amenable to specific interventions, in addition to the general anxiety problems for which he was originally referred. In addition the Beck Depression Inventory suggested that Colin was bordering on mild depression, while the psychiatrist had excluded depression from his diagnosis. As therapy progressed this score decreased dramatically (see Fig. 7.9), and the behavioural and cognitive interventions would seem to have fulfilled a preventive role, with regard to the onset of a depressive episode.

One important aspect remains to be discussed. The model described demonstrates a highly systematic approach to care, that has a wide application in nursing, but it is equally well applied in other disciplines, such as psychology and social work. It is not a model unique to nursing, so is it accurate to describe it as a nursing model?

Certainly, the cognitive-behavioural model offers a theoretical framework to nurses, and can help them to organise their thinking and practice in an orderly and logical way. It deserves a place alongside the other models of nursing, as long as it is made clear that it is not only a model for nursing, but a multi-disciplinary model as well (Fig. 7.13). There are a number of similarities between the cognitive-behavioural model and other specifically nursing models, such as the Roy Adaptation model (Roy, 1980) and the Crisis model (Hawkins, 1983).

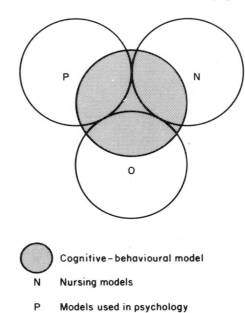

Fig. 7.13 Diagrammatic representation of the association between the cognitive-behavioural model, nursing models and models of other disciplines

Management aspects

The cognitive-behavioural model has been shown to be the treatment of choice in a wide range of conditions. Specific post-registration courses exist to train nurses in the application of the model, and an increasing number of Health Authorities are recognising the benefits of employing behavioural nurse therapists. All new skills tend to be guarded initially by those in possession of them and some elitism has developed in behavioural psychotherapy, where the assumption has been made that only those nurses who have completed long, clinical training can initiate behavioural and cognitive strategies. However, I believe that if a model has been shown to be effective, it should be disseminated as widely as possible. It is refreshing to see that the trend is towards sharing the model with a wide range of nurses. Barker and Wilson (1985) stated that

> The behaviour therapy nursing model can be expressed through a highly sophisticated nurse specialist: perhaps someone who has a need to develop in this direction. The model can also be expressed through basic nursing care. Nurses can use our model to meet basic needs, such as the acquisition of continence or the development of eating skills. The model can be deployed at all stages in between. In this sense the model is a catholic one, for both staff and patients. (p.34)

The trend towards disseminating behavioural skills is illustrated in the high behavioural component in the 1982 RMN syllabus, and the involvement of behavioural nurse therapists in the teaching and supervision of community psychiatric nurses.

To conclude, the cognitive-behavioural model of care has much to offer some people, and something to offer virtually everyone. One does not need to have a psychiatric illness to suffer from a problem that can be relieved by the application of the model.

It can be applied wherever psychological factors are involved in illness, however physical the symptoms may seem. To nurses, the cognitive-behavioural model offers a framework on which to build an empirically derived set of plans for action. For clients it demands an active involvement in decision making, rather than passive implementation of decisions about care made by other professionals.

References

Agras WS, Kazdin AE & Wilson GT 1979 *Behavioural Therapy: Toward an Applied Clinical Science.* WH Freeman & Co, San Francisco.

Arrick C, Voss J & Rimm DC 1981 The relative efficiency of thought stopping and covert assertion. *Behaviour Research and Therapy*, **19**: 17–24.

Bandura A 1969 *Principles of Behaviour Modification.* Holt, Rinehart & Winston Ltd, Eastbourne, Sussex.

Barker PJ 1985 *Patient Assessment in Psychiatric Nursing.* Croom Helm, London.

Barker J & Fraser D 1985 *The Nurse as Therapist: A Behavioural Model.* Croom Helm, London.

Barker PJ & Wilson L 1985 New wine in old bottles. *Nursing Times*, **81**, 39: 31–34.

Beck AT 1976 *Cognitive Therapy and the Emotional Disorders.* International Press, New York.

Beck AT, Rush AJ, Shaw BF & Emery G 1980 *Cognitive Therapy of Depression.* John Wiley & Sons, Chichester.

Bennun I 1980 Obsessional slowness: A replication and extension. *Behaviour Research and Therapy*, **18**: 595–598.

Bird J, Marks IM & Lindley P 1979 Nurse therapists in psychiatry: Development, controversies and implications. *British Journal of Psychiatry*, **135**: 321–329.

Black A 1974 The natural history of obsessional neurosis. In *Obsessional States*, HR Beech (Ed). Methuen & Co Ltd, London.

Brooker C 1984 The differences between community psychiatric nurses and nurse therapists. Paper presented at King's Fund Centre conference: *Nurse Therapy and Community Psychiatric Nursing: Developing Roles*, 17 Jan.

Burns D 1980 *Feeling Good.* Morrow, New York.

Cade B 1980 Strategic therapy. *Journal of Family Therapy*, **2**: 89–99.

Capstick N 1975 Clomipramine in the treatment of true obsessional state. A report on four patients. *Psychosomatics*, **16**, 1: 21–25.

Cawley R 1974 Psychotherapy and obsessional disorders. In *Obsessional States*, HR Beech (Ed). Methuen & Co Ltd, London.

Clarke D, Sugrim I & Bolton D 1982 Primary obsessional slowness: A nursing treatment programme with a 13-year-old male adolescent. *Behaviour Research and Therapy*, **20**: 285–292.

Ellis A 1962 *Reason and Emotion in Psychotherapy.* Lyle Stuart, New York.

Emmelkamp PMG & Kwee KG 1977 Obsessional ruminations: A comparison between thought stopping and prolonged exposure in imagination. *Behaviour Research and Therapy*, **15**: 441–444.

Farrington A 1983 Obsessive compulsive disorder. *Nursing Mirror*, Aug, 17, (vii–viii).

Foa EB & Tillmans A 1980 The treatment of obsessive-compulsive neurosis. In *Handbook of Behavioural Interventions – A Clinical Guide*, EB Foa & A Goldstein (Eds). John Wiley & Sons, Chichester.

Foa EB 1979 Failure in treating obsessive-compulsives. *Behaviour Research and Therapy*, **17**: 169–176.

Frankl VE 1960 Paradoxical intention: A logotherapeutic technique. *American Journal of Psychotherapy*, **14**: 520–535.

Gelder M 1986 Cognitive and behavioural therapies. In *An Introduction to the Psychotherapies*, S Bloch (Ed). Oxford University Press, Oxford.

Hawkins JW 1983 A developmental model: The crises model. In *Nursing Models: Analysis and Evaluation*, JA Thibodeau (Ed). Wadsworth Health Sciences Division, California.

Kanfer FH & Saslow G 1965 Behavioural analysis: An alternative to diagnostic classification. *Archives of General Psychiatry*, **12**: 529–538.

Keen J 1982 The behavioural model. *Medical Education (International) Ltd*, pp. 71–75.

Kirk JW 1983 Behavioural treatment of obsessional-compulsive patients. *Behaviour Research and Therapy*, **21**, 1: 57–62.

Lazarus RS 1971 *Behaviour Therapy and Beyond*. McGraw-Hill Book Co, London.

Lazarus RS 1973 Multimodal behaviour therapy: Treating the 'BASIC ID'. *Journal of Nervous and Mental Diseases*, **156**, 6: 404–411.

Lazarus RS 1985 *Casebook of Multimodal Therapy*. The Guilford Press, London.

Lindley P, Marks I & McCaffery F 1984 National follow-up of nurse therapists. Paper presented at King's Fund Centre conference: *Nurse Therapy and Community Psychiatric Nursing: Developing Roles*, 17 Jan.

Lombardo TW & Turner SM 1979 Thought stopping in the control of obsession ruminations. *Behaviour Modification*, **3**, 2: 267–272.

Mahoney M 1974 *Cognitive and Behaviour Modification*. Ballinger, Cambridge, Massachusetts.

Marks IM, Bird J & Lindley P 1978 Behavioural nurse therapists 1978: Developments and implications. *Behavioural Psychotherapy*, **6**: 25–36.

Marks IM, Hallam RS, Philpott R & Connolly JC 1975 Nurse therapists in behavioural psychotherapy. *British Medical Journal*, 19 July, **3**: 144–148.

Marks IM, Hallam RS, Connolly JC & Philpott R 1977 *Nursing in Behavioural Psychotherapy: An Advanced Clinical Role for Nurses*. Royal College of Nursing, London.

Marks IM & Mathews AM 1979 Fear questionnaire. *Behaviour Research and Therapy*, **17**: 264.

Marks IM & Waters HM 1984 Nurse therapy in primary care. Paper presented at King's Fund Centre conference: *Nurse Therapy and Community Psychiatric Nursing: Developing Roles*, 17 Jan.

Martin GL 1982 Thought stopping and stimulus control to decrease persistent disturbing thoughts. *Journal of Behavioural Therapy and Psychiatry*, **13**: 215–220.

Meichenbaum D 1977 *Cognitive Behaviour Modification*. Plenum, New York.

Mercer S 1985 Obsessional-compulsive disorder. *Nursing Times*, **80**, 34: 34–37.

Meyer V 1966 Modification of expectations in cases with obsessional rituals. *Behaviour Research and Therapy*, **4**: 272–280.

Parkinson L & Rachman S 1980 Are intrusive thoughts subject to habituation? *Behaviour Research and Therapy*, **18**: 409–418.

Paykel E, Klerman G & Prusoff B 1976 Personality and symptom patterns in depression. *British Journal of Psychiatry*, **129**: 327–334.

Rachman S 1974 Primary obsessional slowness. *Behaviour Research and Therapy*, **12**: 9–18.

Rachman S 1976 The modification of obsessions: A new formulation. *Behaviour Research and Therapy*, **14**: 437–443.

Rachman J & Hodgson RJ 1980 *Obsessions and Compulsions*. Prentice-Hall, Englewood Cliffs, New Jersey.

Rimm DC & Masters JC 1979 *Behaviour Therapy. Techniques and Empirical Findings*. Academic Press, London.

Roy C 1980 The Roy Adaptation model. In *Conceptual Models for Nursing Practice*, 2nd Ed. JP Riehl & C Roy (Eds). Appleton-Century-Crofts, New York.

Salkovskis PM & Warwick HMC 1985 Cognitive therapy of obsessive compulsive disorders: Treating treatment failures. *Behavioural Psychotherapy*, **13**: 243–245.

Sher KJ, Frost RO & Otto R 1983 Cognitive deficits in compulsive checkers: An explorative study. *Behaviour Research and Therapy*, **21**: 357–363.

Simon D & Axford T 1983 Something extra. *Social Work Today*, **15**: 3.

Stern R 1978 *Behavioural Techniques: A Therapist's Manual*. Academic Press, London.

Tryon GS 1979 A review and critique of thought stopping research. *Journal of Behavioural Therapy and Psychiatry*, **10**: 189–192.

Turner SM, Hersen M, Bellack AS & Wells KC 1979 Behavioural treatment of obsessive-compulsive neurosis. *Behaviour Research and Therapy*, **17**: 95–106.

Wilde J, Lee D & Axford T 1985 All in the family. *Nursing Times*, **81**, 18: 30–31.

Wolpe J 1958 *Psychotherapy by Reciprocal Inhibition*. Stanford University Press, Stanford.

Yates AJ 1970 *Behaviour Therapy*. John Wiley & Sons, London.

8

Care plan for an overactive person, using Johnson's Behavioural System model

Blair Collister

This chapter explores the application of Johnson's (1980) Behavioural System model in the care of a 32-year-old man admitted to hospital in a hyper-active state.

Literature on the problem of hyperactivity and its nursing management is reviewed to provide the rationale for an approach based on systems theory. The theory is then used in the assessment and identification of patient problems, and a care plan for the patient's first week in hospital is discussed.

Overactivity

Overactivity may occur as a feature of several psychiatric disorders, including mania, schizophre-nia and agitated depression. However, it is difficult to establish a useful definition of the phenomenon which would serve as a yardstick for patient assessment and problem statements. Descriptions of overactivity as a clinical manifestation of mania for the most part reflect that of Sim (1981), who begins a section headed *Hyperactivity* with the statement 'His energy may appear superhuman...' (p.331), and goes on to describe the bizarre activities of a patient whom the author had known.

The value of such descriptions for nursing assessment is questionable. On the one hand they appear more salacious than objective, and on the other hand offer little in the way of an operational baseline or norm by which to discriminate between what is and is not over- or hyperactivity. However, they do imply that hyperactivity is recognised in relation to what is a *normal* pattern of activity for that person, and it is inferred that the problem is recognised in an individualised way.

Another aspect of these descriptions of over-activity concerns the way in which the patient's behaviour is said to affect the social audience, and in particular the response which the behaviour evokes in staff. Thus adjectives such as 'annoying', 'upsetting' and 'wearing-out' are common (Ackner, 1964; Sim, 1981).

However, from a nursing perspective, Wilson and Kneisl (1983) view hyperactivity as one example of disordered *motivation*. Motivation prompts individuals to action, and may be variously viewed as a drive, a need or an instinct, depending on the theory of human behaviour being used to explain the nature of motivation.

Thus regression, withdrawal, impulsive be-haviour, ambivalence and hyperactivity all have as a common element disintegration of motivation.

Hyperactivity is described as

an increase, in the rate of activity. It may include emotional lability and flight of ideas.
(Wilson and Kneisl, 1983: p.412)

It is suggested that the increase referred to in this description is in comparison with what is normal for the particular individual, and it includes reference to mood and thought processes as well as be-haviour. Since the fundamental cause is related to motivation, it is recognised that the overactive patient is not in control of his activity.

With regard to a rationale for nursing interventions in the care of the overactive patient, there is little in the way of research-based literature to support nursing action. Non-research literature reflects an earlier description of nursing care priorities offered by Ackner (1964). In this, the nurse's attention is directed to the need to establish a balance between allowing the patient freedom whilst avoiding nuisance to others; to providing a quiet environment; to discouraging visitors and preventing contact with the outside world. For the patient who is acutely hyperactive, the nurse is directed to the need to maintain nutrition, prevent the patient harming others and preventing exhaustion.

More recently, similar principles are indicated by Wilson and Kneisl (1983) in their suggested rationale for regulating hyperactivity. They describe the verbal interaction between a nurse and a hyperactive patient, and point to the nurse's attempt to minimise external stimuli and avoid disruption to other patients whilst maintaining unobtrusive observation of the patient. Moreover, throughout their discussion, Wilson and Kneisl highlight the nurse's therapeutic use of self, and indicate the ways in which the nurse's interactions are patient-centred and goal directed.

However, even though nurses hold such patient-centred values it may be that other priorities supervene. For example, Street (1982) investigated the priority which psychiatric nurses ascribed to nurse–patient interaction over routine care and physical tasks. The findings of this small-scale study indicated that, when subjects were interviewed

> ... nurse–patient interaction was generally given high priority whereas routine or physical care activities were ranked as less important. (p.26)

The researcher went on to observe the subjects going about their nursing work and

> ... observed very little correlation between priorities expressed in the interviews and observation of the actual work. Routine administrative tasks appeared to be most important and a high proportion of the day was spent in the ward office. (pp.26–27)

Although Brooking (1986) points out several limitations of this study, it is suggested that it

reflects the findings of earlier work by Altschul (1972) and Cormack (1976).

It may be that nurses do have a patient-centred perspective but other aspects of the situation claim their attention when caring for individuals. In particular the need to maintain stability in the social environment of the ward emerges as the highest priority. As a consequence, nurses experience difficulty in putting patient-centred approaches into practice and these take second place. Such a view is supported by accounts of nursing care such as that of Hosker (1983) in which the effects of the admission of an excited patient on the social environment are described, and care is directed to minimising the ensuing disruption.

Thus, a constellation of elements relating to the care of overactive patients are identified in the literature.

These include:

(a) the need to maintain a stable social environment;
(b) the need to balance freedom with supervision and observation;
(c) the need to avoid overstimulating the patient;
(d) the need to ensure that the patient receives adequate food and rest.

These elements – stability, balance, stimulation, intake of food, and rest – reflect concepts central to systems theory including homeostasis, input and output, and conspire to suggest that a nursing approach based on general systems theory may be of value in the care of the overactive patient.

Choosing an appropriate model

In an article discussing an individualised approach to planning care in psychiatric nursing, Altschul (1977) identifies three principal approaches which may be adopted. These are:

1   activities of daily living;
2   the problem solving process;
3   systems theory applied to nursing care.

Altschul suggests that, because of the complexities of the situation in which the psychiatric nurse interacts with the patient, the first two are inadequate. This is because they do not encompass all the variables which may affect the patient, the nurse and the interaction between them.

This view reflects the work of such writers as von Bertalanffy (1966, 1967, 1976), who examine the consequences of increasing the size of organisations, industries and the products and services they provide. One consequence of this increase in size is that the study of problems within such systems becomes more difficult because of size and the number of different aspects which may need to be examined.

It is as a result of such systems problems, von Bertalanffy suggests, that a new discipline emerged – that of general systems theory. It is suggested here that it is not merely size which generates such complexity. As knowledge about the natural world increases, so the realisation develops that things are not as simple as they seem. It is a case of 'the more you learn the less you know'. Hence, as nursing knowledge increases through systematic enquiry, questioning practice, and research, so nurses become aware of the complexity of the job of nursing. Thus any theoretical approach may be of value to nurses if it helps them to make sense of, and predictions about, nursing, and facilitates the testing of hypotheses and establishing of relationships.

General systems theory

A system is a whole with interrelated parts, in which the parts each have a function and the system as a whole has a function. Systems operate in relation to both the immediate and distant environment through the processes of *input, transformation, output and feedback.*

Disorganisation is always present in a system because of adjustments resulting from input, and because of the energy loss associated with transformation and feedback. However, systems tend towards balance, or equilibrium, to promote the survival of the whole.

Interaction between the system and the environment takes place through the *boundary* of the system. *Open* systems show the greatest contact and interplay with the environment, and all living systems are classed as 'open'. Natural phenomena may be studied by considering them at hierarchical levels of complexity. Thus simple systems may be regarded as subsystems of more complex systems.

The *structure* of a system refers to the arrangement and nature of its organisation, and the term *function* denotes the interaction between the parts. It should be noted that systems theory is directed to the *interaction* between the parts, and not to the function of the parts themselves. When a system is in equilibrium it is impossible to discriminate the function of one part from another.

Stress is resisted (and equilibrium maintained) by:

1 ignoring the existence of an external stressor; or
2 activating homeostatic forces; or
3 achieving a new state of equilibrium.

Johnson's Behavioural System model

Johnson (1968, 1980) applied systems theory to nursing by viewing the person as a behavioural system. She accepts the notion that a system is a whole which functions by virtue of the interdependence of its parts.

Johnson (1980) defines human behaviour as 'overt actions in response to internal or external stimuli'. She suggests (1968) that human behaviours can be grouped according to the function they serve. Based on these groupings, she identifies seven subsystems. These are: affiliative, dependency, ingestive, sexual, eliminative, aggressive-protective and achievement. To this list, Grubbs (1980) has added an additional behavioural subsystem, which she terms restorative. It should be noted that this addition is not accepted by Johnson (1980: p.214).

Each subsystem has five structural components: goal, set, choice, action and sustenal imperatives.

The *goals* of each subsystem are indicated in Fig. 8.1, and it is suggested that these help to clarify the reasoning behind Johnson's functional grouping of human behaviours. Also, attention is drawn to the labels attached to each behaviour. Some have both a definitive and an associative

Fig. 8.1 Behavioural subsystem goals

SYSTEM/SUBSYSTEM	GOAL
Person (total system)	**Survival and adaptation**
Ingestive (subsystem)	To take in a substance, object or information that the individual perceives to be lacking.
Eliminative (subsystem)	To release waste products, excess or non-functional matter ($\rightarrow$ tension release).
Dependency (subsystem)	To seek help to attain another goal.
Sexual (subsystem)	To procreate, and collective survival.
Affiliative (subsystem)	To belong or associate with others in some form of specific relationship.
Aggressive/protective (subsystem)	To protect self, others or property from real or imagined harm.
Achievement (subsystem)	To master/control self and environment so as to obtain a desired object, position or need.
Restorative (subsystem)	To maintain the energy balance in the system through redistribution of energy.

meaning, so that, for example, *ingestion* refers to the ingestion not only of food but also of information and air. Thus any behaviour which is directed to 'taking things in' would be classified as ingestive and could include breathing, reading, listening and touching as well as eating and drinking.

The term *set* refers to the consistency of response to a particular stimulus. Responses may occur as a matter of habit, or be modified through experience. *Choice* refers to the idea that there may be a variety of possible responses to a particular stimulus, and the person selects the best from these alternatives.

Behaviour which can be observed is termed *action*. This observable behaviour may or may not occur. There is no half-way house, it either happens or it does not happen.

The term *sustenal imperatives* has been criticised on the grounds that it is unfamiliar and obscure. However, it is suggested that the term *need* is a useful substitute, since sustenal imperatives are necessary for the survival of the system. For behaviour to continue it must be protected from harmful stimuli, nurtured through having adequate input and stimulated to continue its development.

Deficiency in sustenal imperatives threatens the function of the subsystem and the survival of the system as a whole, and it is suggested that sustenal imperatives serve as the focus for the identification of patient problems and the selection of appropriate nursing action.

Grubbs (1980) suggests that a person becomes a patient in need of nursing when there is a loss of order and predictability in the behavioural system. She classifies the kind of behavioural discrepancies which may occur under three headings.

1 *Disorderly* – Regression, or failure to carry out usual routines.
2 *Purposeless* – Repetitious, goalless actions, or directed to a goal which does not benefit.
3 *Unpredictable* – Differs from what may be expected.

In the case of 'expected' behaviour, Grubbs suggests that the present behaviour may be:

(a) compared with past behaviour;
(b) compared with common patterns;
(c) compared with responses described in the literature.

In discussing the notion of 'normal' behaviour, Grubbs suggests that the boundaries of 'normal' are set by society, but that professionals tend to impose a narrower band of what may be 'acceptable'. This point has particular significance for psychiatric nurses.

To take a simple example, it is not unusual to find long-stay wards where the routine requires patients to get up, washed and fully dressed, and to make their beds before partaking of breakfast. To be regarded as 'normal' by nurses, patients must adhere to this regime. Yet the same nurses may not readily adapt to such a regime themselves and may have family members who would challenge such expectations. A similar argument concerning the inconsistency between social and professional definitions of 'normal' could be advanced for things like shaving, wearing make-up, having a bowel movement every day, drinking three litres of fluids every day, or making cups of tea at irregular times.

In some instances it appears that the definition of 'acceptable', if not of 'normal', is refined for the convenience of professional health carers rather than for the therapeutic benefit of patients and their discharge from care or treatment. This assertion relates to nursing situations generally, and not just to the circumstances of this particular model. It is therefore necessary to be precise when describing behaviour, and especially when stating that a particular aspect of a person's behaviour is abnormal.

Loss of order and predictability in a person's behaviour is recognised, then, as behavioural discrepancy, and is classified as outlined above. Having recognised such discrepancies, the nurse then seeks to identify the nature and cause of those which are amenable to nursing action.

Loss of order and predictability may occur either:

(a) within one subsystem (insufficiency, discrepancy); or
(b) between two or more (incompatibility, dominance).

Nursing action is directed to providing the sustenal imperatives necessary for the functioning of the subsystem(s) showing behavioural discrepancies.

Nursing intervention may be any one of four types.

1 *Restricting* – Imposes limits/external controls on behaviour.

2 *Defending* – Protects by preventing damage.
3 *Inhibiting* – Nurtures by preventing ineffective response.
4 *Facilitating* – Nurtures/stimulates to help cope with demands.

Statements of nursing action should include two elements indicating the nature of the nursing intervention. The first indicates which subsystem and which structural part is the focus of nursing action, and the second indicates the mode of intervention, for example to alter the set, broaden choices, modify the action or alter the goal.

The model in practice

The writer had established contact, and a good relationship, with ward staff prior to the work undertaken for this care study. Before the implementation of the Johnson Behavioural System model in the care of the patient selected for this study, a series of informal teaching sessions had been held to familiarise staff with the elements of the model.

These sessions also included discussion of the general use of models in nursing practice and the relationship between nursing models and the nursing process. Existing nursing documentation was used for the nursing history and assessment, and adapted by the addition of headings reflecting the behavioural subsystems.

Grubbs advocates the use of a two-stage assessment process. The goal of the first level assessment, which is general but thorough, is to decide whether or not a problem amenable to nursing intervention exists. If such a problem does exist, then the second level assessment is carried out. This two-stage assessment is reflected in the accompanying nursing history and care plan. The patient's background and the circumstances leading to admission are summarised in Fig. 8.2.

The admission record (Fig. 8.3) includes relevant biographical and other data, and a summary of the observations which indicated that a problem was present. The subsequent second level assessment, shown in Fig. 8.4, was carried out during the 24 hours following admission and

Fig. 8.2 Background information and admission circumstances of John T

John T is a 32-year-old telephone engineer. He was divorced a year ago, his wife and 2 children had moved to another part of the country and John had moved in to live with his parents. He had one period of hospital inpatient treatment 3 years ago, about the time of his marital separation, and shortly after that had left British Telecom to join a private telephone company.

His parents describe him as a quiet, shy man, modest in his behaviour. After he had been made redundant, John became even quieter than usual, and spent most of each day alone in his room. He then began to behave in an erratic manner and became (for him) very talkative and overactive. His parents recognised the signs from his previous episode, and called their general practitioner. The GP prescribed chlorpromazine, which was in addition to Priadel which had been prescribed for the previous 3 years.

However, John's behaviour continued to concern his parents, because he was eating and sleeping poorly, becoming more overactive around the home and talking about various plans for work which his parents felt that he had no hope of bringing to fruition. They contacted their GP again, and after another visit to the home the GP contacted the CPN team.

The Community Psychiatric Nurse visited John and his parents at home and, as a consequence of the obvious strain which John's parents were experiencing and in view of the fact that John had not taken any of his medication for 3 weeks, arranged admission for him.

the care plan was drawn up at that time. This care plan addresses the high priority problems present at the time of admission. Depending on the progress made in resolving these problems, a further care plan addressing other problems, which would by then have assumed high priority, would be drawn up. The reasons for this are twofold.

Firstly, it is the author's experience that problems which assume a low priority at the time of admission (for example family disharmony, non-compliance with medication regimes, and maladaptive coping strategies) tend not to be dealt with adequately at any time during a patient's stay in hospital. These problems may well be much more significant in the long-term, are often the more intractable and demand more ingenuity on the part

of the nurse in their resolution. Thus, once life-threatening problems are resolved, little attention is directed to the further care required and few, if any, individualised therapeutic interventions are employed.

Secondly, once the acute phase of disturbed behaviour has subsided, and the nurse has been able to develop a therapeutic relationship with the patient, then the patient can have the opportunity to participate in his care. This participation may not have been possible initially, but now the patient can validate problems, share in goal identification and agree the amount and nature of nursing and patient action. Drawing up a second care plan therefore provides the opportunity for patient participation and ensures a review of the priority of problems.

Turning to the care plan (Fig. 8.5) the problems are presented in relation to what was thought to be the appropriate behavioural subsystem. These subsystems were listed in alphabetical order on the second level assessment. Consequently, when decisions were made about nursing action and the action written into the care plan, it was found that problems later on the list had been addressed by action designed to help with problems listed earlier. In order to avoid repetition, these actions were cross-referenced on the care plan, and it is suggested that this experience serves to illustrate the focus on the interaction of the behavioural subsystems.

It is interesting to note that, for the problems identified within the restorative subsystem, no original nursing action is specified and the nurse is referred to five other subsystems. This may be interpreted in one of two ways. It could be that the classification 'restorative' is superfluous, and since the problems so classified are addressed under other categories of behaviour then Johnson's refutation of this subsystem is supported.

Alternatively, and particularly for the sort of patient problem under discussion, it may be that the behaviour classified as 'restorative' is the main focus of nursing intervention. This could be so particularly for the stage represented by this care plan. Indeed, had the list begun with this subsystem, then almost all the nursing actions noted on the care plan could have been placed into this category. Thus the behavioural classification res-

Fig. 8.3 Admission record

Name: John N T	**Date of birth:** 22.5.54 Age 32
Address: Moorside, Northtown	**Marital status:** Divorced
Home circumstances: Lives with parents	**Community services:** **GP** Dr A N
	CPN visit F R 24.7.86

Next of kin: Parents, S/A

Occupation: Telephone Engineer

Religion: C/E Non-practising

Admission circumstances

Date: 24th July 1986. Made redundant 1/12 ago. Increasingly disturbed since then. Previous admission 1983. Divorced one year ago. Has not taken Priadel for 3/52. Seen by GP referred to CPN. Admission arranged.

Admission assessment

(First level)

Arrived accompanied by parents. Jovial, garrulous rapid speech, very restless. Appears unkempt. Recent weight loss.

Difficult to sustain conversation. Says he is here to 'help out'.

Signature: ....

Date: .... 24th July 1986 ....

---

torative, rather than being redundant, emerges as a key element.

Evaluation

In evaluating the use of Johnson's model in practice, attention is directed firstly to the implications for staff education which arose from the preliminary teaching sessions.

It was found that the general idea of systems theory was understood by ward staff, and that the concepts were easily grasped and accepted. Two particular misgivings were resolved following discussion. The first of these was the idea of 'behaviour', which was associated with behavioural psychology and which some staff had been involved in through the medium of operant conditioning and token economy. Considerable explanation and

discussion was required to establish the idea of 'behaviour' in this context as 'observable action'. Although some principles of behaviour therapy are incorporated in nursing action, in particular that of reinforcement, this is by no means the only mode of action. Nursing care therefore goes beyond mere behaviourism.

The second problem centred on the general idea of behavioural subsystems. Staff felt that, having been exhorted to take a holistic approach to individual patients, they were now expected to 'dismantle' patients into discrete elements. Two approaches were taken in addressing this. The first was to re-examine systems theory and to emphasise the interaction between subsystems as the main focus, rather than the subsystems in isolation. The second, on a more philosophical level, was to discuss the application of systems theory in

Fig. 8.4   Second level nursing assessment

Nursing assessment (Second level) Nurse: B C	
Achievement	Recently made redundant. Speech rapid, almost incoherent. Pacing corridor and room. Informs staff of his own extraordinary abilities. Asks to be informed of condition of all other patients with whom he has contact. Does not sustain goal-directed activity, e.g. washing, dressing, eating, conversation. Fully aware of environment.
Affiliative	Recent deterioration in relationship with parents. Overbearing in social exchange, ignores the reaction of others. Speaks of concern for others, although to no purpose.
Aggressive/protective	Not hostile or aggressive. Overconfident about his abilities to overcome risks to physical and psychological well-being. Becomes jovially irritable when limits set. Insensitive to the needs of other patients. Disinhibited in expressing wishes.
Dependency	Resists dependent relationship with staff. Rationalises admission to hospital as 'here to help cure the others'. Ignores threats to security.
Eliminative	Immodest language when referring to elimination. Normal micturition. Constipated. Perspiring profusely.
Ingestive	Reacts to almost all stimuli in the immediate environment – sensory overload. Drinks 2.5 l in 24 hours. Food neglected. Medication discontinued 3 months ago.
Restorative	Has not slept since admission (24 hours). Neglects hygiene, continuous activity – pacing, exercises. Over-expends energy – potential exhaustion. Inappropriate response to potential hazards – false beliefs about his own abilities.
Sexual	Divorced – wife and two children have moved away. Unable to assume appropriate parental and spouse roles. Disinhibited and flirtatious in conversation with female staff and patients.

psychiatry, and to examine the values underpinning this approach. Particular reference was made to the work of von Bertalanffy in this context.

Von Bertalanffy (1967) suggests that systems may be useful in situations where multivariate components are found. This is especially so when to expect simplicity and clarity is unreasonable, and when the situation cannot adequately be dealt with by 'traditional' science, whether, for example medical (Collister, 1986) or social (Parsons, 1975). Further, von Bertalanffy (1976) has identified two trends in general systems theory. The first is a mechanical approach which has given rise to cybernetics, computerisation, flow charts and regulation by feedback. It appeared that nurses' misgivings rested on such a perception of the behavioural systems model.

However, von Bertalanffy (1976) has identified a second trend, which he terms the organismic-humanistic approach. This allows scope for free will and individuality, and the system plays an active part in the dynamics of the situation rather than being a passive victim of inputs, feedback and control.

Based on this, von Bertalanffy has developed certain principles.

1 Non-reductionism: this emphasises the interaction between subsystems and the function of the system as a whole. This is in contrast to isolating the function of different parts each from the other.
2 The system (person) is active in maintaining balance, rather than a passive victim of inputs, feedback and control.
3 The emphasis is on human, not mechanical systems.
4 There is a trend to higher organisation. This suggests that interactions between systems, as parts of higher systems, are the focus and is the corollary of the non-reductionist view.
5 Human and supra-biological values are introduced into science. Thus humanistic principles, and ethical and moral values influence decision making.

Fig. 8.5 Care plan

Date	Subsystem/ problem	Goals	Review date	Action	Evaluation
25.7.86	*Achievement* Unable to sustain goal directed behaviour in carrying out activities of living.	Sustain actions to wash, dress and eat.	3 days.	Supervise and encourage washing, bathing, dressing. Meals in room. Stay with patient. Encourage to eat and drink.	28.7.86 Responding to supervision and encouragement. 29.7.86 Eating in dining room. 28.7.86 Eating most of each meal.
		Maintain adequate hygiene and nutrition.	1 week.	Give assistance where necessary.	
25.7.86	*Affiliative* Alienates others through overbearing manner and lack of sensitivity.	Decrease frequency of the behaviour which others finding upsetting.	3 days.	Distract if behaviour offends. Remove from presence of others if behaviour persists.	28.7.86 Others upset less frequently.
		Increase awareness of effects of behaviour on others.	3 days.	Explain effects of behaviour on others. Encourage other patients similarly.	28.7.86 Not fully aware of effects on others – continue distraction/ explanation. Review 31.7.86.
25.7.86	*Aggressive/protective* Ignores risks to physical and psychological well-being.	Recognise potentially harmful situations.	1 day.	Protect from injury. Explain/indicate hazards. Restrain from hazardous behaviour.	26.7.86 Perception of risks still inappropriate. Review 3.7.86
		Modify response appropriate to environmental hazards.	1 week by discharge.	Accompany patient off ward. Role model, e.g. working in ward kitchen, crossing road.	30.7.86 Behaviour more appropriate to hazards, but still reckless at times. No injury sustained.

Fig. 8.5   (continued)

Date	Subsystem/ problem	Goals	Review date	Action	Evaluation
25.7.86	*Dependency*				
	Inappropriate perception of hospital admission.	Accept need to remain in hospital.	Daily until discharge.	Ask patient to advise staff if he wishes to leave ward (or hospital)	26.7.86 Misperception of admission continues.
		Maintain independence.	Up to and following discharge.	Accompany in grounds/outside hospital.	27.6.86 Accepts need of staff advice and to be accompanied.
		Recognise events which brought about hospital admission.	By discharge.	Discuss admission events. Discuss usual coping strategies. Discuss future plans.	30.7.86 Discusses admission circumstances freely – more accurate perception of admission events. 4.8.86 Recognises inappropriate perceptions and states the need to continue medication.
25.7.86	*Eliminative*				
	Disinhibited when expressing emotions.	Will exercise restraint when expressing emotions.	3 days.	See Affiliative.	28.7.76 Use of immodest language decreasing.
	Constipated.	Achieve bowel movement.	Daily.	Give aperient. Monitor result. Give high fibre diet and 3 l fluid per day. See also Achievement.	26.7.86 Bowels opened.
		Re-establish normal bowel habit (every other day).		Monitor/ask patient to advise.	4.8.86 Adequate diet taken. Usual bowel habit re-established.

Fig. 8.5 (continued)

Date	Subsystem/ problem	Goals	Review date	Action	Evaluation
25.7.86	*Ingestive* Oversensitive to external stimuli.	Avoid excessive stimuli. Reduce distractability.	Daily. 1 week.	Nurse in single room. Minimise light/noise/distraction when conversing. Involve in ward tasks requiring short attention span. See also Achievement and Eliminative.	26.7.86 Reluctant to remain in room. Restless, pacing.
		Re-establish medication regime as prescribed.	Daily to discharge.	Give medication as prescribed.	27.7.86 Medication given as prescribed. 30.7.86 Medication continued.
	Inadequate dietary intake.	Take part (at least) of each meal. Re-establish normal diet. Weight gain of 4 lb.	Daily. 1 week.	See Achievement and Eliminative.	27.7.86 Eating some of each meal with supervision and encouragment. 1.8.87 Weight 10 st 6 lb (gain 3 lb).
25.7.86	*Restorative* Insomnia	Protect from harm.	Daily.	See Aggressive/protective.	26.7.86 Night sedation as prescribed.
	Overactive, potential exhaustion.	Reduce overactivity.	Daily.	See Dependency.	Slept 2–5 am. Remains restless and overactive.
		Maintain adequate rest and sleep.	Daily.	See Ingestive.	27.7.86 Occupied for part of day in kitchen. Slept for 4 hours; 2–6 am.
		Restore normal sleep pattern.	1 week.	See Affiliative and Eliminative.	1.8.86 Slept 6 hours. Much more settled during day.
25.7.86	*Sexual* Unable to resume previous spouse/parent roles.	Find appropriate outlets for sexual expression.	By discharge and subsequently.	See Affiliative Dependency. Discuss previous psycho-sexual patterns.	Continues.

However, it may be that Johnson's focus on the person as the system limits the value of her model to the practice of psychiatric nursing. In many instances the person (patient, nurse, family member) is part of a larger social system, and it is this larger system which becomes the focus of nursing interventions. Examples of such social systems include group work with patients, the social milieu in a ward, and the patient's family. Elaboration of the model would be necessary to encompass such situations.

Aggleton and Chalmers (1984) have pointed out that nursing models are the product of logical development, and have emerged from a 'body of understanding often referred to as the human sciences'. Johnson's model fits this description, especially if von Bertalanffy's principles and their implicit values are incorporated in the application in practice.

Johnson (1980) indicates the relevance of the knowledge of various behavioural and biological sciences to her model. Whilst acknowledging that a great deal of work remains to be done to establish a body of *nursing* knowledge, Johnson makes no explicit reference to the skills of the nurse, particularly in establishing and maintaining a therapeutic relationship with the patient. Thus, whilst the model reflected in this care plan appears adequate, it may have limited applicability in other situations. In particular it may be that the social environment is inadequately conceptualised. Lobo (1985) notes that 'definitions of the concepts are so abstract that they are difficult to use'. However, abstract definitions may be useful in that they allow practitioners to make their own interpretations in adopting a model. On the other hand the energy and imagination needed for such mental gymnastics may be more fruitfully directed to nursing practice, with the practice framed within a model more appropriate to an interpersonal (rather than intrapersonal) approach.

Conclusion

The experience of using Johnson's Behaviour System model has provided lessons of both a general and a specific nature.

Working with the nurses on the ward confirmed the need to involve them from the outset in any proposed change. In the case of nursing models this means exploring nurses' perceptions of the concepts involved in the model and providing assistance to help their understanding. If concepts such as 'stress' 'behaviour' or 'self-care' are familiar, it is important not to assume that the meaning ascribed to them by nurses is the same as their meaning or significant in nursing models.

The second point to be confirmed was that the usefulness and limitations of a particular nursing model may only become evident when the model is used in practice. Although this point may seem obvious it is nevertheless important. Unrealistic optimism based on the perceived utility of a model may lead to a failure to anticipate and deal adequately with practical problems, whereas uninformed rejection may lead to a self-fulfilling prophecy such that the practical advantages of a model are ignored. All involved should therefore be prepared to modify not only the documentation, for example, but also their own perceptions. Such a situation has developed through the author's involvement in the use of Johnson's model.

The limited view of the nurse–patient relationship referred to earlier was not obvious at the onset. Although this is perceived as a weakness of the model in the writings of Johnson, it may also be an advantage in practice since it offers the opportunity to apply other ideas, possibly through the elaboration of other tenets basic to Johnson's model. For example, the interpersonal and social aspects of a person's situation may be addressed by reference to the dependency, affiliative and achievement subsystems. However, it would be the *interaction* between these subsystems which would be of primary concern, and not the function of each in isolation from the others. In this way the first of the 'Bertalanffy principles', outlined above, would be applied in a non-reductionist approach.

Finally, the repetition which began to emerge when writing the care plan gave impetus to thinking about ways of streamlining the documentation. On a less concrete level it points to the need for more work on identifying the significance of the various behavioural subsystems in the identification and resolution of patient problems. Thus the experience of working with others in the use of this model not only provided a wealth of practical information, but also helped to highlight issues of a more abstract nature which will require additional thought and investigation in practice.

References

Ackner B 1964 *Handbook for Psychiatric Nursing*, 9th Ed. Balliere Tindall, Eastbourne.

Aggleton P & Chalmers H 1984 Defining the terms. *Nursing Times*, **80**, 36: 24–28.

Altschul A 1972 *Patient–Nurse Interaction: A Study of Interaction Patterns in Acute Psychiatric Wards*. Churchill Livingstone, Edinburgh.

Altschul A 1977 The Nursing Process in Psychiatric Care. *Nursing Times*, **73**, 36: 1412–1413.

Bertalanffy L von 1966 General systems theory and psychiatry. In *American Handbook of Psychiatry Vol 3*, S Arieti (Ed). Basic Books, New York.

Bertalanffy L von 1967 *Robots, Men and Machines*. Braziller, New York.

Bertalanffy L von 1976 *Introduction to Health Research: The Systems Approach*, HH Werley, A Zuzich, M Zajkowaski & AD Zagornik (Eds). Springer, New York.

Brooking J (Ed) 1986 *Psychiatric Nursing Research*. John Wiley & Sons, Chichester.

Collister B 1986 Psychiatric nursing and a development model. In *Models for Nursing*, B Kershaw & J Savage (Eds). John Wiley & Sons, Chichester.

Cormack DF 1976 *Psychiatric Nursing Observed*. Royal College of Nursing, London.

Grubbs J 1980 An interpretation of the Johnson Behavioural System model for nursing practice. In *Conceptual Models for Nursing Practice*, 2nd Ed, JP Riehl & C Roy (Eds). Appleton-Century-Crofts, New York.

Hosker N 1983 Excitement in the ward. *Nursing Mirror*, **157**, 13: 39–40.

Johnson DE 1968 One conceptual model of nursing. In *Behavioural Systems and Nursing*, JR Ager (Ed). Prentice-Hall, Englewood Cliffs, New Jersey.

Johnson DE 1980 The behavioural system model of nursing. In *Conceptual Models for Nursing Practice*, 2nd Ed, JP Riehl & C Roy (Eds). Appleton-Century-Crofts, New York.

Lobo ML 1985 Dorothy E Johnson. In *Nursing Theories*, 2nd Ed, J George (Ed). Prentice-Hall, Englewood Cliffs, New Jersey.

Parsons T 1975 The sick role and the role of the physician reconsidered in health and society. *The Millbank Memorial Fund Quarterly* Summer 1975, pp.257–278.

Riehl JP & Roy C 1980 *Conceptual Models for Nursing Practice*, 2nd Ed, Appleton-Century-Crofts, New York.

Ruddock R (Ed) 1972 *Six Approaches to the Person*. Routledge & Kegan Paul, London.

Sim M 1981 *Guide to Psychiatry*, 4th Ed. Churchill Livingstone, Edinburgh.

Street CG 1982 An investigation of the priority on nurse–patient interaction by psychiatric nurses. In *Psychiatric Nursing Research* (J Brooking 1986). John Wiley & Sons, Chichester.

Wilson HS & Kneisl SL 1983 *Psychiatric Nursing*, 2nd Ed. Addison-Wesley, London.

9

Care plan for an anxious person, based on Cawley's Levels of Psychotherapy

Susan Ritter

In this chapter, a multidisciplinary approach to the care of an anxious patient is described. The model described is that of the Levels of Psychotherapy (Cawley, 1976) used in conjunction with the nursing process and primary nursing in an acute general psychiatry ward of a teaching hospital. Professor Robert Cawley developed his classification of the Levels of Psychotherapy in the early 1970s following 'a feasibility study for a controlled trial of a type of psychotherapy' (Candy *et al.*, 1972). Its use as more than just a frame of reference was an interactional process between all disciplines, including the ward's other consultant, Dr Murray Jackson, who shares responsibility for the general psychiatry beds and is a practising psychoanalyst. The integration of the classification into the ward's policies and procedures evolved over a number of years. For this reason the interpretation of the model presented here differs from that of Faugier and Reilly (1986).

Levels of Psychotherapy

Cawley emphasises that 'the classification is of techniques not treatment programmes' (Cawley, 1976). The term 'level' does not imply a system which values one level over another, but represents the attempt to find a neutral term in order to facilitate the tailoring of a given approach to an individual patient. Interpersonal and interactional techniques appropriate to each level or category are identifiable and can be taught, learned, practised

and applied as required by the care plan for the patient.

The assumptions of the nursing care defined by this model may be traced via Sundeen *et al.* (1985); the psychosocial nursing practised at the Cassell Hospital (Barnes, 1968) and the Henderson Hospital (Rapoport *et al.*, 1960); the numerous accounts of work at Chestnut Lodge (Searles, 1965); and Peplau (1952). Interwoven strands include Sullivan's (1953) interpersonal theory of psychiatry which underpins Peplau's exposition of nurse–patient relations, and Meyer's (1913) socially-based psychobiological psychiatry.

Elements of the model

The definitions here are taken from the ward's professional operating procedures.

1 *P1 psychotherapy* in its widest sense is co-extensive with the doctor–patient or nurse–patient relationship. It is required in *all* clinical situations.

2 *P2 general psychotherapy* is required by all psychiatric patients. This includes aspects of treatment elsewhere described as supportive, directive, non-directive, focal, client-centred and distributive. The common factor is the development and use with therapeutic intent of a *professional* relationship whose form and content are tailored to the needs and reality situation of the patient as perceived by the

patient and the nurse, doctor or other therapist, and to the time and facilities available. The objectives are as diverse as the patient's problems and there is no unitary theoretical basis. All members of the multidisciplinary care team need to be competent in the practice of general psychotherapy.

3 *P3 formal psychotherapy* depends on the establishing of a transference relationship within which the therapist offers to the patient a series of interpretations relating the transactions within this relationship to present and past experiences. It identifies and interprets unconscious conflicts and in so doing dismantles defences and evokes anxiety in the short term, with the aim of resolving it more permanently.

4 *P4 behavioural and cognitive psychotherapy* comprises a group of techniques derived from experimental psychology. Behaviour therapy is a treatment for observable (dysfunctional) behaviour which is based on a range of experimental evidence from the fields of learning theory and cognitive and social psychology (Gelder, 1983). Cognitive therapy is directed towards helping clients to identify and restructure the ways in which they think about themselves and their interactions with other people and their environment.

Theoretical background

The background assumption for the nursing use of this model derives from Kuhn (1970), and declares that the discipline of nursing is in a prehistory phase, moving towards the status of a Kuhnian community of scientific professional groups producing and validating scientific knowledge, but still with some way to go. The model tries to make sense of observable phenomena in a hospital ward, to replicate nursing activities over time, to examine the consequences of these activities and to provide a schema for explanation, supervision and teaching. No claims are made for its logical harmony nor for its axiomatic basis, and it will be noted, for instance, that reliance on the concept of the unconscious is an anomalous feature (Feyerabend, 1978). The medical model is not rejected but is disregarded where it is irrelevant to nursing care. Diagnosis is seen as the business of the doctors, who may use nurses' observations, but who understand that nurses fulfil an independent role in the multidisciplinary care team (Martin, 1976; DHSS, 1980).

It is assumed that every part of a nurse's interaction with a patient is potentially therapeutic or non-therapeutic, whether they are waiting in a cafeteria queue together or medication is being given. Primary nursing is the means by which nurses are assigned to individual patients and work closely with each other in a containing framework. The monitoring and supervision of nurse–patient interaction can be achieved only in the context of individual patient assignment. It has been demonstrated that nurses defend themselves against the stress of working intensively with sick and damaged people and against recognition of their own dependency needs. Defences used include transient work allocations, and busy task-oriented activity (Winnicott, 1949; Main, 1957; Menzies, 1960; Burnham, 1966; McGilloway, 1976; Gunther, 1977; Manthey, 1980). The complex relationships between nurses and patients produce inevitably strong emotional responses that are not easily understood. Primary nursing allows nurses to develop a relationship over time, to recognise that they can respond with equal intensity to patients' feelings, and to use their professional colleagues to help them step back from a relationship. Timely help and advice from associate nurses and supervisors can prevent nurses from proceeding with interventions that may lead to harm for them as well as for the patient (Balint, 1957).

The model of the Levels of Psychotherapy attempts to demystify as well as emphasise aspects of the interpersonal process, while specifying the areas of psychotherapeutic work which require specialist training and knowledge. In texts and articles written by nurses, use of psychoanalytic concepts such as denial, projection, transference, identification or interpretation, demonstrate an often uncritical interest in the practice of psychotherapy. These concepts tend not to be used to the advantage of dependent and vulnerable inpatients, but as a means of distancing nurses from them – 'the retreat from the patient' (Kubie, 1971). Similarly, the apparent incompatibility of psychoanalytic psychotherapy and behaviour therapy derives from the attitudes of some of the people using them rather than from their inherent properties. The Levels of Psychotherapy model provides a framework within which to use measures for the nursing application of techniques such as active listening, consensual validation, negotiation, problem-solving or record-keeping. Patient outcomes may then be compared with measurable factors in their relationships with nurses (Stanton and Schwartz, 1954; Cormack, 1975; Barker, 1982, 1985).

Relationship to other nursing models

The Levels of Psychotherapy model attempts to follow Chapman's advice (1976) to spell out its specific origins in the behavioural and biological sciences. It shares with Peplau (1952) and Sundeen *et al.* (1985) a debt to the concept of symbolic interactionism: that a person's individuality is defined by his response to the expectations of other individuals in his environment (Mead, 1934). It shares with King (1981), Neuman (1980), and Sundeen *et al.* (1985) a caution in defining the recipient of nursing care, as well as in defining nursing care itself. It does not set out to define the nature of man although it is recognised that aspects of so-called humanistic psychology are contained in Peplau's conceptual framework (1952), and that Rogers (1980), Roy (1980) and Johnson (1980) use the nature of man as a starting point. The Levels of Psychotherapy model is well suited to the dynamic nature of the nursing process, and to an inter-system model of nurse–client interaction (King, 1981; Artinian, 1983).

Care study

Jen is a teacher in her late twenties. She works in a large comprehensive school where she became interested in pastoral work as a result of teaching disadvantaged children. She herself has had intervals of psychiatric treatment since the age of six,

and entered formal psychotherapy in 1983. She was referred and accepted for five-times weekly psychoanalysis in 1984. At about the same time Jen split up with her fiancé. Over the next few months she began to use street drugs and to experience what she described as panic attacks. Her teaching timetable was reduced, but she offered to resign as she felt less and less able to cope. Her resignation was not accepted, and she started to take anti-depressants, prescribed by her GP. Eventually, Jen's therapist referred her to be admitted to hospital because she feared that Jen would seriously harm herself. On admission Jen described her increasingly chaotic lifestyle and her growing reluctance to leave her house, use public transport, and leave her analyst's rooms at the end of her sessions. She used the words 'panic' and 'anxiety' to describe her state but also felt that she had many serious and long-standing difficulties in forming and sustaining relationships. Her disrupted upbringing had resulted in long separations from her now divorced parents. She felt that she was being helped by the psychotherapy and felt committed to continuing. Her therapist wished to continue the therapy and arranged to continue seeing Jen in the ward, because Jen's cessation of travelling on public transport effectively prevented her from attending her therapist's rooms.

Anxiety

Jen's bewilderment about herself and her anxious feelings reflect the mystery of anxiety, its nature and origins. While she was able to attribute some of her panic to travelling on buses or trains, she also experienced it in the absence of any cause that she could identify. What made it more difficult for both Jen and her friends was that she rarely looked anxious, rarely demonstrated any of the signs that are usually accepted as indicating anxiety. The consultant who admitted her hoped that she could be helped quite quickly with her specific fears about travelling, but he was less hopeful about what would be possible in the short term to help Jen with her generalised anxiety.

Rachman and Wilson (1980) argue that anxiety can be seen as comprising three systems: the patient's own account, his behaviour, and physiological changes. Similarly Marks and Lader (1971) suggest that these systems may combine in up to nine main patterns, with some patterns deficient in one or two of the systems or components. For instance, Jen complained of feeling anxious, behaved in an agitated way, but experienced no physiological changes. The current state of theory about the kind of generalised anxiety experienced by Jen in addition to her specific fears of travelling offers little guidance for clinical management (Tyrer, 1984). In recent years, patients like Jen have tended to be treated with anxiolytic measures, with drugs such as benzodiazepines which produce physiological dependence; or with relaxation techniques, with little diminuition of their anxiety. In contrast, behavioural treatments of phobias rely on anxiogenic measures – exposure to what is feared.

The more specifically a care team can determine responsibility for aspects of treatment the more chance there is of identifying what works and what does not. Ideally the anxiety evoked during a session is allayed by the end of it through the skills of the therapist. However, 'uncovering' psychotherapies, no matter how soundly based, may evoke a degree of anxiety for longer periods than the patient can bear without having to employ emergency defensive measures such as damaging acting-out. The team must contain the distress as best they can, but the uncertainties about the efficacy of interventions, combined with Jen's increasingly urgent expressions of anguish, seriously threatened the nurses' ability to work together and with other members of the team.

Assessment

Level P1 psychotherapy requires attention to the safety of the patient, as well as to the strategies for nurses and patients to get to know each other. The nurse's duty of care is the foundation of the nurse–patient relationship and so the primary nurse is responsible for drawing up a safety care plan which precedes any assessment (Fig. 9.1). Unlike the care plans drawn up later, in order to conduct the assessment and to carry out the nursing care planned as the result of the assessment, the objective of the safety care plan is not negotiable.

Jen's compliant response to her safety care plan aroused some reservations in her nurses, combined with puzzlement about her anxiety and the absence of physiological signs. Jen's primary nurse, in the next phase of establishing their level P1 relationship, agreed with her an assessment programme using a series of care plans designed to assess Jen's anxiety in different circumstances (Fig. 9.2).

The primary and the associate nurses together were responsible for the progress notes which included the nursing assessments and summaries,

Fig. 9.1 Safety care plan

Probem	Objective
At present Jen has ideas of harming herself and feels she might want to run away.	Jen will remain free from serious self-injury both on and off the ward for the next five days.
What Jen will do	
1 Jen will refrain from leaving the ward alone. 2 Jen will tell her nurses if she has any thoughts of harming herself or running away. 3 Jen will negotiate with one of her nurses when she wants to leave the ward.	
What (Jen's nurses) will do	
1 Accompany Jen if she wants to leave the ward. 2 Arrange to spend at least thirty minutes with Jen each shift in an activity of her choice. 3 Let Jen know where they will be if she wants to talk with them.	
Outcome	**Evaluation**
Jen has not harmed herself or run away during the past five days.	Jen and the nurses have carried out their agreed actions. The plan is renewed for a further five days.

Fig. 9.2   Assessment care plan

Need	Objective
Jen needs to assess her levels of anxiety on and off the ward over the next seven days.	Jen will maintain anxiety ratings on and off the ward over the next seven days.

What Jen will do
1   Fill out her anxiety rating charts as discussed with her nurses.
2   Give them to her primary nurse in seven days time.
3   Discuss them with her nurses.
4   Let her nurses know when her anxiety rises above a level she can tolerate.

What (Jen's nurses) will do
1   Discuss Jen's rating charts with her.
2   Participate with Jen in an activity of her choice if she feels her anxiety is above a level that she can tolerate.

Outcome	Evaluation
Jen completed her charts (see Fig. 9.3).	Jen and the nurses carried out their agreed actions apart from Jen not needing to implement No 4. Jen will keep the charts for another seven days.

the shift-by-shift objectives not contained in the care plans, process records of interactions, and Jen's own notes, summaries and diaries. The results of the rating scales (Fig. 9.3) were placed on a graph so that the fluctuations could be seen at a glance and compared with the nursing notes which described the events and activities which formed the background to the assessment. Jen's self-ratings were compared with those of the nurses in order to see how their perceptions differed from hers. The process recordings of their interactions provided the means of assessing the rapport developing between Jen and her nurses and the quality of their level P1 relationship.

After four weeks, during which the ward doctor and occupational therapist had been conducting their own assessments, the first case conference or ward round of Jen's admission was held. Her primary nurse presented the results of the nursing assessment and Jen was interviewed. The consultant did not wish to interfere with the psychotherapist's work, but felt that he could identify clearly Jen's claustrophobia and agoraphobia which he explained afterwards in terms of object relations and the severe childhood deprivation experienced by Jen (Jackson and Jacobson, 1985).

Plan

The team decided that their priority was to help Jen to start travelling alone again in order for her to

Fig. 9.3   Anxiety chart

Activity	Anxiety rating 1–10						
Sitting in the lounge	7	6	7	7	5	6	6
Going to the bus stop	6	6	7	6	4	6	7
At the bus stop	7	6	6	8	5	7	7
Going back to the ward	5	5	6	5	4	6	5
Back in the ward	6	7	5	6	4	3	3
Making morning coffee	5	5	6	5	4	6	5
In the canteen lunch queue	6	6	7	6	4	6	7
Day	S	M	T	W	T	F	S

undertake her formal psychotherapy while living at home, and having started work again. Jen said that this was what she wanted. Levels P1 and P2 psychotherapy were to be used to help Jen to move into the world outside the hospital and to concentrate on her analysis as the way of understanding her disturbing but apparently meaningless tensions. A risk was identified of forming a special relationship with Jen in which she tried fruitlessly to find a way of gaining peace and freedom from her fears. Progress in her therapy would inevitably provoke episodes of tension and fear as understanding and insight grew (Jackson *et al.*, 1986). Jen would be tempted to look for solutions that were anxiolytic, that took away her anxiety. Hence her abuse of street drugs. It seemed that the main question for the team now was to identify when it would be practicable to expect Jen to live with her feelings at home, since her job was at risk and the financing of her house depended on her teaching salary.

During the next phase of Jen's admission her nurses concentrated on a graded exposure programme of travelling (see Fig. 9.4), starting with trips to the local shopping centre, progressing to the West End and finally to her therapist's rooms. The programme was a routine level P2 application

of behavioural techniques (Barker, 1985). Meanwhile the ward doctor started an anxiety management programme with Jen, supervised by a behaviour therapist (Matthews, 1986). This was a level P4 package of cognitive strategies, relaxation and behavioural techniques. After six weeks Jen was travelling alone on buses. After seven weeks she was able to travel as far as her therapist's rooms, including times after 6 pm. Peplau (1952) suggests that four phases (orientation, identification, exploitation and resolution) in nurse-patient relationships can be identified. Clinical experience with mentally disordered patients such as Jen suggests that nurses' relationships with them tend to fluctuate in ways that Peplau's stages do not fully explain, tempting though the structure is. The nursing assessment of Jen required her to participate fully in the process of identifying her needs and problems, so that the nurse was not solely a resource person as in Peplau's orientation phase. Jen's nurses sometimes actively directed aspects of her review of what led to her admission, sometimes adopted a non-directive approach, so that Peplau's identification phase is not an exact description of what happened. And as will be described, the apparent exploitation and resolution (in Peplau's terms) by Jen, using her relationship with her

Fig. 9.4 Example of an exposure programme care plan

Need	Objective
Over the next next seven days Jen needs to travel as far as (her therapist's) rooms on a bus in preparation for travelling there on her own.	Jen will make two bus journeys with (her nurse), and two on her own over the next seven days.
What Jen will do	
1 Plan her journeys. 2 Negotiate her plans with (her primary nurse). 3 Make the journeys as planned. 4 Keep a record of her anxiety ratings.	
What (Jen's nurses) will do	
1 Negotiate Jen's plans with her. 2 Accompany her on two of the journeys. 3 Discuss her anxiety ratings with her.	
Outcome	**Evaluation**
Jen completed all four journeys despite moderate anxiety.	Jen is also experiencing generalised anxiety and finds it difficult to identify the cues for it. She is prepared to continue the travelling programme.

nurses, led into areas where formulae would not work. The Levels of Psychotherapy model provides an exact image of the nurse using techniques and approaches according to the immediately expressed needs of the patient, sensitive to the fluctuations in the patient's ability to accept what is on offer. Jen's nurses moved to the next stage of planning with as few preconceptions as possible.

For a while it looked as though Jen would soon be leaving hospital. But as her specific fears of travelling decreased she would achieve a journey and would go out again to buy alcoholic drinks, returning to the ward intoxicated. She burnt herself with cigarettes and took various over-the-counter drugs. Her behaviour aroused hostility in some staff and sympathy in others. Some staff felt hostile towards her therapist for apparently exacerbating Jen's behaviour, and for maintaining the privacy round the therapy.

Weeks dragged on. Jen's primary nurse emigrated to work abroad. Jen and the new primary nurse found it difficult to form a working relationship. Jen would not agree care plans with specific objectives and her nurses felt unable to help Jen find some activity in which she could feel rewarded. Despite her therapist's assurances that progress was continuing, the nurses found it difficult to accept that their apparently unnecessary role was useful in any way, a feeling also belied by their extensive notes which documented their persistence in maintaining their level P2 relationship with Jen. Jen portrayed her therapist to them as incompetent, and, they suspected, portrayed them in the same way to her therapist. She complained of terrible panic, emptiness and feeling out of control (Jackson and Pines, 1986).

An in-group and an out-group such as those described by Main (1957) formed round the issue of tranquillising medication. Both Jen's therapist and the consultant favoured Jen's starting medication. They saw Jen as gripped by unbearable anxiety, linked to her past childhood deprivation and aroused now at the end of each session when she had to leave her therapist. Some of the nurses and other staff saw Jen's behaviour as a challenge to be resisted. Although the readiness to use medication is an essential component of level P2 psychotherapy, some of the staff persuaded them-

selves that 'talking therapy' was the only way of achieving success and that intervention with medication, especially if it was requested by Jen, represented failure.

The cycle of events which is set in train when a group of staff become divided over the care of a 'special patient' can, according to Main (1957), be redirected in ways that are helpful to the patient; but only if the staff are prepared to undertake an often painful process of self-examination and self-disclosure in group settings. Their discussions must be led by someone with the skills and knowledge necessary to help colleagues towards understanding of the ways in which their emotional responses to a patient are shaped unconsciously both by the patient's past experiences of caring figures, and also by their own past. The meetings and discussions will be difficult for staff to tolerate, especially as people develop at different rates and in different ways and are likely always to be at different stages of progress towards understanding. Particular tolerance is required by the nurses, along with a willingness to see each other, themselves and the patient in different ways. The conflict between the staff over Jen's medication was gradually resolved as the nurses and other staff recognised how the strength of their support, opposition or indifference for medication derived from emotional responses to Jen and those most closely involved with her care. Her primary nurse, in particular, saw how the falling off in productive care planning with Jen appeared to re-enact the inadequacies of caring figures in Jen's past.

Medication was prescribed and Jen began to take it regularly. Later she negotiated a care plan with her nurses in an attempt to control her feelings of rage against them when her therapist went on holiday (Fig. 9.5).

Evaluation

After five weeks Jen stopped taking medication and restarted the exposure programme. At the time of writing she has a discharge date for almost fourteen months after admission. She remains fragile and anxious. Her story demonstrates how level P3

Fig. 9.5 Nursing care plan

Probem	Objective
Jen has violent thoughts towards nurses prior to (her therapist) going on holiday.	Jen will refrain from allowing these thoughts to become actions over the five days.

What Jen will do

1 Inform her nurses when she feels violent.
2 Try to discuss her difficulties with the nurses.
3 Ask for chlorpromazine when she thinks she needs it.

What (Jen's nurses) will do

1 Ensure that Jen knows where they are if she wants to talk to them.
2 Discuss Jen's difficulties with her.
3 Arrange for Jen to have chlorpromazine when she asks for it.

Outcome	Evaluation
Jen refrained from any violence.	Jen has been talking to her nurses and also, but not always, takes 50 mg chlorpromazine. Continue the plan for a further five days.

psychotherapy or psychoanalysis with seriously disturbed patients may not be feasible without the back-up of the other levels. Additionally, each level may be feasible, but used individually fails to address the whole person. In Jen's case, the inputs from levels P1, P2 and P4 are insufficient without the psychodynamic dimension of level P3, used not only as a method of treatment but also to inform the strategies used by the nurses in their care of Jen.

Conclusions

This approach to nursing with the psychotic or severely personality-disordered patient offers the hope of applying psychoanalytic psychotherapy to a proportion of such very disturbed people. The psychoanalytically informed character of the work rests on the assumptions that unconscious mental processes exist and may be extremely potent; that so-called symptoms and abnormal behaviour have meaning; and that the attempt to understand and to communicate something of that meaning to the patient in an effective way can be of considerable help to the patient (Jackson, 1986).

The ability of nurses to apply these assumptions to their nursing care derives from the careful discrimination between the Levels of Psychotherapy, which ensures that the skills and knowledge appropriate to each level are taught, learned and absorbed under the close supervision and direction of a charge nurse whose authority is clearly delegated through the primary nursing system. For the multidisciplinary care team as well as for the trained and learner nurses within it, the Levels of Psychotherapy model contributes to a means of genuine cooperative professional work. For the nurses, it represents a greatly increased development of their practice, both therapeutic and defined in terms of the constituents of nursing care. Soundly based in the same educational philosophy which informs the training of mental nurses, it is supported in a framework of management providing the supervision necessary for them confidently to accept the accountability for their individual patient care. It is detailed and comprehensive enough when used with primary nursing both to predict and to evaluate accurately the resource needs of a ward at any given time, and provides both the tools and the subject for research into the nature and efficacy of psychiatric nursing.

References

Artinian B 1983 Implementation of the inter-system patient-care model in clinical practice. *Journal of Advanced Nursing*, 8: 117–124.
Balint M 1957 *The Doctor, his Patient and the Illness.* Pitman Medical, London.
Barker PJ 1982 *Behaviour Therapy Nursing.* Croom Helm, London.

Barker PJ 1985 *Patient Assessment in Psychiatric Nursing.* Croom Helm, London.

Barnes E (Ed) 1968 *Studies in Psychological Nursing.* Tavistock, London.

Burnham DL 1966 The special problem patient: Victim or agent of splitting? *Psychiatry*, **29**: 105–122.

Candy J, Balfour FH, Cawley RH *et al.* 1972 A feasibility study for a controlled trial of psychotherapy. *Psychological Medicine*, **2**: 345–362.

Cawley RH 1976 Assumptions and Preconceptions about Psychotherapy. Paper delivered to the Association of University Teachers of Psychiatry, Conference on *The Teaching of Psychotherapy*, 24 Sept.

Chapman C 1976 The use of sociological theories and models in nursing. *Journal of Advanced Nursing*, **1**: 111–127.

Cormack D 1975 The nurse's role in psychiatric institutions (1). *Nursing Times*, **71**, 51, Occasional Paper: 125–128.

Cormack D 1975 The nurse's role in psychiatric institutions (2). *Nursing Times*, **71**, 52, Occasional Paper: 129–132.

DHSS 1980 *Report of the Working Group on Organizational and Management Problems of Mental Illness Hospitals.* DHSS, London.

Faugier J & Reilly S 1986 Taking time to talk. *Nursing Times*, **82**, 18: 52–54.

Feyerabend P 1978 *Against Method.* Verso, London.

Gelder MG 1983 Anxiety and phobic disorders, depersonalization and derealization. In *Handbook of Psychiatry*, M Shepherd & O Zangwill (Eds). Cambridge University Press, Cambridge.

Gunther MS 1977 The threatened staff: A psychoanalytic contribution to medical psychology. *Comprehensive Psychiatry*, **18**: 385–397.

Jackson M 1986 A psychoanalytical approach to the assessment of a psychotic patient. *Psychoanalytic Psychotherapy*, **1**, 2: 11–22.

Jackson M & Jacobson R 1985 Psychoanalytic hospital treatment: The application of psychoanalytic principles in psychiatry. In *Psychiatry: The State of the Art Vol 4*, P Pichot (Ed). Plenum, New York.

Jackson M & Pines M 1986 The borderline personality: Concept and criteria. *Neurologia et Psychiatria*, **8**, 6: 54–57.

Jackson M, Pines M & Stevens B 1986 The borderline personality: Psychodynamics and treatment. *Neurologia et Psychiatria*, **9**, 1: 66–88.

Johnson D 1980 The behavioural systems model for nursing. In *Conceptual Models for Nursing Practice*, JP Riehl & C Roy (Eds). Appleton-Century-Crofts, New York.

King I 1981 *A Theory for Nursing.* John Wiley & Sons, New York.

Kubie LS 1971 The retreat from patients. *Archives of General Psychiatry*, **24**: 98–106.

Kuhn TS 1970 *The Structure of Scientific Revolutions.* University of Chicago Press, Chicago.

McGilloway FA 1976 Dependency and vulnerability in the nurse–patient situation. *Journal of Advanced Nursing*, **1**: 229–236.

Main T 1957 The ailment. *British Journal of Medical Psychology*, **30**, 3: 129–145.

Manthey M 1980 *Primary Nursing.* Blackwell, Oxford.

Marks I & Lader M 1971 *Clinical Anxiety.* Heinemann, London.

Martin AJ 1976 Duty of care. *Nursing Times*, **72**, 36: 1379.

Matthews A 1986 *Anxiety Management Training.* Unpublished treatment schedule, Department of Psychology, St George's Hospital, London.

Mead GH 1934 *Mind, Self and Society.* University of Chicago Press, Chicago.

Menzies I 1960 (1970) *The Functioning of Social Systems as a Defence Against Anxiety.* Tavistock Publications, London.

Meyer A 1913 (1948) *The Common-Sense Psychiatry of Dr Adolph Meyer.* McGraw-Hill, New York.

Neuman B 1980 The Betty Neuman health-care systems model: A total person approach to patient problems. In *Conceptual Models for Nursing Practice*, JP Riehl & C Roy (Eds). Appleton-Century-Crofts, New York.

Peplau H 1952 *Interpersonal Relations in Nursing.* GP Putnam's Sons, New York.

Rachman SJ & Wilson GT 1980 *The Effects of Psychological Therapy.* Pergamon Press, Oxford.

Rapoport RN *et al.*, 1960 *Community as Doctor.* Tavistock Publications, London.

Rogers M 1980 Nursing: A science of unitary man. In *Conceptual Models for Nursing Practice*, JP Riehl & C Roy (Eds). Appleton-Century-Crofts, New York.

Roy C 1980 The Roy Adaptation model. In *Conceptual Models for Nursing Practice*, JP Riehl & C Roy (Eds). Appleton-Century-Crofts, New York.

Searles HS 1965 *Collected Papers on Schizophrenia and Related Subjects.* The Hogarth Press, London.

Stanton AH & Schwartz MH 1954 *The Mental Hospital.* Basic Books, New York.

Sullivan HSS 1953 *The Interpersonal Theory of Psychiatry.* WW Norton, New York.

Sundeen SJ, Stuart GW, Rankin ED & Cohen S 1985 *Nurse–Client Interaction – Implementing the Nursing Process*, 3rd Ed. CV Mosby Co, St Louis.

Tyrer P 1984 Classification of anxiety. *British Journal of Psychiatry*, **144**: 78–83.

Winnicott DW 1949 Hate in the countertransference. *International Journal of Psychoanalysis*, **30**, 2: 69–74.

10

Care plan for an aggressive person, based on Peplau's model of nursing

Gary Rix

This chapter explores the nurse's use of interpersonal skills in a secure environment. Using Peplau's (1952) model, it demonstrates the process through which the nurse is encouraged to share the patient's perception of his situation and to identify the reasons underlying his behaviour.

The care plans provide the overall goal of care and are used as a framework to guide each interaction with the patient.

The discussion examines the situation in which a patient's problem attracts contrasting interventions from medical and nursing staff and the nurse's dilemma in such a situation.

The aggressive patient

The literature on violence in hospitals is not extensive but what there is produces fairly consistent findings. Most violent incidents are trivial in nature with the victim suffering little or no physical injury. A small number of patients are usually responsible for a large proportion of incidents. All the research is plagued by lack of an agreed definition of what constitutes a violent incident; definitions range from verbal threat to actual assault. Drinkwater (1982) gives a comprehensive review of the literature on the subject of violence.

Hodgkinson *et al.* (1984) carried out a survey of violent incidents in a London hospital. They found that nurses were the main victims (94%), with over 50% of assaults being caused by under 20% of the patient population. They found schizophrenics to be the most aggressive diagnostic group. In looking at increases in violence over time they found increases took place in admission and locked intensive care wards.

In an earlier study Fottrell (1980) found that 10% or less of patients actually behaved violently. He found that schizophrenic patients were consistently the most violent but reminds us that this is due to 'schizophrenia' being the most common diagnosis. Other more anecdotal accounts of violence within secure settings are provided by Campbell and Mawson (1978) in their description of life on a ward at John Connelly Hospital. Again they highlight the fact that some patients are more violent than others, and these people they label 'special cases'. The authors make a plea for a small lockable area in a ward to manage such individuals, since they carried out assaults of a different order resulting in individuals being 'badly beaten up'.

The need for such security was questioned by Cobb and Gossop (1976) in their study of a locked ward at the Maudsley Hospital. They quote Bell (1955) who claimed that

> the ideal nurse–patient relationship is not reached until doors are unlocked

and Mandlebrote (1958) who stated

> keys and locked doors do much to destroy both staff–patient relationship and perpetuate anxieties and insecurities felt towards one another.

This question of security and its effect on relationships is discussed below.

Weaver, Broome and Kat (1978) and Weaver *et al.* (1978) produce some interesting findings on behavioural patterns within a secure setting. They assume that the environment and staff expectations are powerful factors in influencing the behaviour of patients. Specifically, they suggest that patients transferred to a locked provision are thought to be unmanageable and disruptive, that the mentally ill are not thought to be accountable for antisocial acts and that nursing attitudes and management practices maintain such behaviour. Behaviours specific to a secure ward are physical assault, repeated abscondings, damaging property and suicidal and self-mutilating acts.

They quote other research (DHSS, 1976; Sommer, 1969; Dabbs, 1971; Emiley, 1975; Paulus *et al.*, 1975) which shows that conditions found in secure units may generate disturbed behaviour. These include lack of privacy, crowding and frustration resulting from being unable to leave the ward. In terms of interpersonal skills the way a nurse approaches a patient may similarly exacerbate rather than alleviate aggressive behaviour.

Lee (1980) in an anecdotal account of the philosophy of care in a special hospital states that nurses assumed that the patient would be violent and therefore would crush any signs of this before it escalated. Insulin therapy seemed to help but in the author's view it was not the insulin that radically altered patients' behaviour but the 'change of environment' and a 'human approach to the individual'. He continues 'hospital life was degrading, inhuman and unnatural and this produced precisely the situation that they (nurses) were attempting to eradicate'.

Lemmer (1979) records in a care study how the aggressive patient is less likely to be popular and less able to form a relationship with a nurse. This view is supported by studies of the attractiveness of patients, including those of Brown *et al.* (1973) and Doherty (1971). Violence can be seen as a response to frustration of needs. Nurses are ideally placed to investigate such needs and move the patient towards verbalising them rather than becoming violent. Lemmer (1979) gives an account of how this approach worked with a patient.

Clack (1963) writes of a study of the way nurses react to aggressive behaviour. She identifies three responses. Firstly the 'counter transference reaction' in which the nurse reacts to her own unresolved difficulties in expressing aggression by setting limits and failing to talk through the situation thus denying any opportunity for learning. In a second scenario labelled 'the pattern of manifest reaction to anxiety' nurses show free-floating anxiety about the aggressive patients. They are unable to do anything and show behaviours such as helplessness, ingratiation, avoidance and a tendency to change the environment for the patient. Such strategies allow no exploration of thoughts or feelings. In the third situation of 'therapeutic nursing intervention' free communication and exploration with the patient, mutual reduction of anxiety and consistent intervention based on theory and observation allow learning to take place for both individuals.

Clack's paper closely follows Peplau's own thoughts on nursing the aggressive patient:

> Permitting the patient to express aggression toward a nurse who listens therapeutically may aid the patient in becoming aware of his feelings and goals.

In Taylor's (1985) study of prisoners at Brixton a fifth of the sample acted on delusions or hallucinations while a further fifth probably did so. Delusions were the most common trigger to violence.

Taylor (1982) discusses the relationship between psychosis and violence. She suggests caution in that such studies are fraught with the problems of diagnosis and definition. Studies concentrate on people who have perpetrated some major violent act such as murder. Taylor observes that

> There is no truly satisfactory epidemiological study which defines a section of the general population and examines the rates of violence and psychosis within it. The chances of an individual psychotic person being seriously violent are probably small. While people with affective psychosis still seem to be at little risk of acting violently toward others, schizophrenics may be at greater risk of criminally violent behaviour than non-psychotics.

Peplau's adaptation of a frustration model of

aggression is attractive as it allows nurses to consider what part they play in frustrating patients' needs and wishes and to move towards a mutual examination of these needs. Peplau states 'when needs are met new and more mature ones emerge'. Nurses in practice need to explore whether this principle bears true.

Peplau's model of nursing

Psychiatric nurses have long struggled for an identity separate from that of other nurses. The nagging question of 'what do psychiatric nurses do?', and what their theoretical basis is for doing it, often throws the profession into confusion. Perhaps a model of nursing that values the nurse–patient relationship and talks of it as a tool for change can go some way toward answering these questions.

Cormack (1973) identified a discrepancy between the prescribed role of nurses and what they actually did as demonstrated in a study of charge nurses. Time spent in interactions with patients was minimal and was then mainly social in nature or enquiring of the patients' state. Similarly Altschul (1972) concluded in her study of psychiatric nurses that

> with the present level of nurses' skill and knowledge it would appear that relationships between nurse and patient were irrelevant to psychiatric treatment.

Towell (1975) asserted that prescriptions about the desirability of nurse–patient interactions had little effect on behaviour. The main objective of interactions was social control.

There is little evidence that things have changed (Duggan and Rix, 1987) and certainly in secure units there is a danger that nurses still adopt a moral retributional model where the nurse as an agent of change is not seen as a viable role (see Baldwin (1983) for fuller discussion).

It is against this background that Peplau offers a framework in which nurses can exercise their potential as educators and facilitators of personal growth.

Peplau's model for nursing is outlined in her book *Interpersonal Relations in Nursing* (1952). The model is grounded in her experience as a nurse educator and practitioner and in theories of personality development. A founding belief is that the chief function of nurses is the maintenance of effective interpersonal relations and transforming nursing situations into learning situations. In order to achieve this the nurse assists the patient in the identification of problematic situations and of personal strengths towards learning and growth. This pre-dates the work of Rogers (1961) who states that change comes through experience in a relationship.

Peplau considers that there are four phases to the nurse–patient relationship. The first, orientation, involves the patient recognising that there is some form of illness that requires the intervention of a professional helper. This is the first step of the learning experience and one that unfortunately many people experience negatively. Usually this is because the focus tends to be on the eradication of symptoms and neglects the feelings and attitudes of the patient.

Nurses can help by providing clarification of problems, and educating when the patient's understanding or knowledge is lacking. The patient needs to achieve a number of objectives in order that learning may occur during this phase. The need to recognise the problem, accept the need for help, recognise that help is available and harness energy toward solving the problem.

In the second phase, identification with those who can help occurs. Peplau states that there are three possible outcomes to this; that the patient proceeds on a basis of participation and interdependence with the nurse, that the patient is isolated from and independent of the nurse, or that there is a helpless dependent relationship.

All of these responses may be experienced and may indeed be necessary, but in this relationship the nurse needs to examine with the patient what his preconceptions of nursing are and to consider her own beliefs about the patient's ability to deal with the problem at hand.

In the third phase the patient exploits the situation in which he finds himself. This involves using the resources at his disposal which will include nurses.

In the final phase the patient's needs are met and

he begins to formulate new goals as he moves toward discharge. If the patient's needs are not met during earlier stages they may be expressed as vague symptoms, such as headaches. The patient now must move toward independence from the nurse and a 'freeing process' occurs as working bonds are severed.

During all of these phases the nurse fulfils a number of roles including stranger, resource person, teacher, leader, counsellor and surrogate mother or sibling.

In the final part of her book Peplau discusses the development of personality and those skills the nurse may need to help the patient achieve this. These are learning to count on others, learning to delay satisfaction, and identifying self.

The model is appealing as it focuses primarily on the relationship between nurse and patient and how it can be used to therapeutic effect. This is particularly relevant to psychiatric nurses who have skills to offer, particularly when the medical model is proving inadequate for those patients whose symptoms will not simply go away and who need help in coping with life and living with long term disability (see Salvage, 1985).

The model, however, makes a number of assumptions that may prove hard to substantiate. Peplau sees man as an organism with needs that, if unfulfilled, create tension and anxiety. The nurse acts to identify these needs and either meet them or help the patient delay fulfilment. This offers an idealistic picture of nursing. Research has shown that nurses are particularly poor at meeting patient needs (Goffman, 1961; Barton, 1959) and may indeed subjugate patients' needs in order to satisfy their own. This is not so much a criticism of Peplau but rather demonstrates the difficulty of implementing her ideas in some hospital environments.

The concerns of a secure unit may require that the fulfilment of patients' needs is postponed for the greater good, particularly when there is a conflict between patient and nurse over such issues as safety. It is usual in such circumstances that nurses cannot live with the anxiety, and move quickly to control the patient so that the ward atmosphere is not disturbed. Peplau's model neglects the social context of nursing and refers only to the interpersonal field, and its use may therefore promote a 'social control' approach.

Other roles the nurse may have then are custodian, gaoler and agent of control.

Peplau's model lays great emphasis on the skills of the nurse as a person and her ability to work with the patient and look critically at her own beliefs and assumptions about the patient. This requires great flexibility on the part of the nurse and an ability to work non-judgementally with people who can often stretch patience and personal resource to the limit. This has implications for nurse education and for nursing practice which, as Menzies (1960) suggests, can be rigid and routinised in the extreme.

Peplau makes a number of assumptions about the patient: that he will have capacity for growth through learning, that he accepts the need for hospitalisation (not always the case when detained against their will under the Mental Health Act), that he wishes to enter into a working relationship with the nurse and that he has the cognitive ability to conceptualise problems and needs. If these conditions are not met then the patient will never move from an unsuccessful orientation phase and the model will not prove helpful. This paints a picture of the nurse as custodian, never moving into a therapeutic relationship with a hostile and unwilling patient.

Care study

John is a 23-year-old man of West Indian extraction. He was born in Leeds and by all accounts had a settled and loving home background. Around his twelfth birthday the family returned to Trinidad but found they could not settle and subsequently returned to England.

On their return John began playing truant from school and got into a number of fights, culminating in his suspension from school for an attack on another pupil and the headmaster. After this he continued his education at home. At the age of 17 he took up a labouring job.

Soon after, John's mother died suddenly. He was the only boy in a home dominated by a mother who was loving and who did a great deal for him, so much so that after her death he needed constant care as he was unable to perform such basic living skills as washing and cooking. The importance of the relationship is also shown by his own admission that he still finds it too painful to discuss. It appears that his mother collapsed at a church service and her condition was thought to be due to 'religious ecstasy'. No medical help was called. She was put to bed and died later in the night. At the funeral John attacked one of the church-goers as he felt they were responsible for her unnecessary death. At this time John became reckless, stating that the worst possible thing had happened to him, and that nothing now could hurt him.

John was dismissed from his employment for his rebellious and anti-authority attitude. In an atmosphere of recriminations at home he assaulted his sister, and when his father was called he threatened him with a knife. John was now abusing a number of drugs: cocaine, heroin, cannabis and amphetamines. Friends described a change in his personality from someone who was clear-headed to being indecisive and muddled.

Some nine months later he was admitted to hospital. There was a six-month history of paranoid ideation and auditory hallucinations. Whether these were drug-induced is uncertain but John stated he had been using only cannabis for 4–5 months prior to admission. At this time he was described as hypervigilant and suspicious. In three incidents he struck other patients or staff and was often verbally aggressive, threatening to beat up nurses who were 'broadcasting' his thoughts. Some of these incidents were thought to be directly triggered by his illness while others were described as a result of his 'aggressive personality'.

John took his own discharge and was at that time symptom free. Soon after this he was arrested for conspiracy to rob. He was subsequently convicted and given a seven-year sentence.

In prison John became ill again. He was suspicious of the way people were looking at him, felt spied on, thought people were talking about him when no one was there and believed others had entered his cell and written racist slogans on the wall. His reaction to this was to threaten other inmates with violence. He was transferred to a hospital wing and there, while on anti-psychotic medication, improved. However, his medication

taking was marked by periods of refusal and, prior to his transfer to a secure unit, was stopped altogether. It was reported that John was unsettled and worried by his anticipated move.

Assessment

Peplau's model, unlike some others, does not provide comprehensive documentation which guides the nurse in her thinking when making an assessment of patient need. It is, in any case, desirable that the nurse should try to understand the world from the patient's point of view and elicit needs or problems from him rather than imposing a rigid conceptual framework. In this way the patient owns the problem and is motivated to construct/conceptualise it in a logical way. There is literature that suggests that such an approach speeds resolution of problems. For the nurse to participate in this process requires skill in listening, conceptualising problems, negotiation and facilitating patients in moving toward resolution. This coming together Peplau terms orientation.

The headings used for care plans in this chapter are partly those adopted by the Bethlem Royal and Maudsley Hospitals. They are meant to provide flexibility in order that any model can be used. This documentation is basically plain paper with the headings: patient's name, primary nurse's name, need/problem, nursing intervention, patient's objectives, nursing intervention and evaluation summary, with spaces for signatures. The format here follows this closely.

When John was admitted to the secure unit he was suspicious and apprehensive. He was accompanied by two prison officers and gave his name as Peter. He was shown to his room and commented that he thought the place would be open and so was concerned that doors were locked as he passed through the unit. Although John had been seen some months previously to be assessed for his suitability for admission, the officers accompanying him were interviewed to ascertain how John had been recently. They stated that for the last two months he had been more relaxed and sociable, less suspicious and hostile towards others and was eating and sleeping well. This they put down to his commencing medication. This had recently been stopped and he had become more restless and anxious about the transfer.

John clearly stated that he did not want to be in hospital because he was not ill. He explained that life in prison had been made difficult for him by the 'screws'. Now he was in hospital he would 'make a go of it'. I explained to John that I was his primary nurse and would be assisting him during his stay.

John's first care plan was written at this time and was later discussed with him. It outlined one area that had been of concern to other professionals and two that John had expressed (see Fig. 10.1).

At this stage violence or aggression were not referred to directly as this had not been a problem in the recent past. At this point the nurse is in the role of resource person and educator helping the patient to orientate to the ward and what it may offer. It is worth noting that John did not accept the

need for such provision. This is a common experience as some prisoners never accept the need for hospitalisation and never regard themselves as patients but as still 'doing time'.

It quickly became apparent that John was suffering from some abnormal experiences. He complained that on a visit from a relative he was having difficulty conversing and concentrating as he could hear voices in the distance. He complained that his bed was moving at night and described vividly how this had happened in prison as well. He said people were making things difficult for him by 'being funny toward me' and 'tormenting and testing me'.

What was most alarming was his interpretation of events and intended reaction to them. He recalled that in prison he had been told the bed moving was a figment of his imagination, and this made him feel like 'slashing him (the doctor) with a knife'. On the ward he swore at people and told them to 'watch themselves' because he felt they were staring at him. He smashed his bedroom chair because he would rather that than hit a nurse for making his bed move. Generally, John put the worst possibly interpretation on people's actions in an attempt to make some sense of the abnormal experiences he was having.

At this point there was a danger that nursing staff and John would become polarised, with nurses laying down the law that violence was not allowed (see Clack, 1963) and becoming ever more restrictive to a man who was already paranoid, hostile and possibly violent and who did not accept the need for hospital admission or that he was ill. The situation now further worsened when John was involved in fights with two other patients.

A breakthrough came when, during a long conversation, John became quite angry that so little had been done about the voices he was hearing. He recalled his previous experience of hospital and stated he wanted some medicine that would 'cure' him. A new care plan was drawn up to capitalise on this move into an identification/exploitation phase. It included specific instructions on how nurses should communicate with him (Fig. 10.2).

The nurses were not directly confronting John with their perceptions of events but rather offering alternative views. Acceptance of these views was

Fig. 10.1   Care plan 1

Problem/need

1   John says he is unsure whether he wants to be here.
2   John says he finds it difficult to establish new relationships and to settle into new places.
3   Others (prison service) are unsure whether John suffers from a mental illness. John states that he is not ill but that others torment him and make life difficult.

Patient objectives

1   John has agreed to talk regularly with his primary nurse about settling into the unit.
2   John has agreed to report to his primary nurse when he feels people are 'out to get' him.

Nursing interventions

1   John's allocated nurse will assist him in settling into the unit by explaining the routine (this will be helped if the allocated nurse is not changed too often).
2   Nurses are to record any evidence of mental disturbance in the nursing record. Particularly:

    (a)   complaints of auditory hallucinations;
    (b)   John stating others are talking about him or making reference to him;
    (c)   accusing others of talking about him;
    (d)   making threats to others.

Fig. 10.2 Care plan 2

Problem/need

1 John feels nurses are persecuting him by ignoring his requests, making life difficult for him on the unit by not letting him sleep, making his bed move and 'tormenting' him.

Patient objectives

1 Rather than threatening or hitting nurses or patients, John will listen to their reasons for their actions/interventions.
2 John will speak to his primary nurse about his perceptions of the unit, particularly when feeling persecuted.

Nursing interventions

1 To communicate clearly and calmly reasons for nursing actions/interventions.
2 If John is violent, to approach him when calm to elicit reasons for his actions.

---

based on trust which was not always present, for example, John: 'The nurses ignore me – they want to torment me. . . .', Nurse: 'Sometimes the nurses are very busy and can't give you as much time as you'd like'.

There was still anxiety about John's potential to harm someone but this receded once medication was commenced and his mental state improved rapidly. He was in better humour, more relaxed, and less troubled by voices. He said that his bed still moved but was not so noticeable and he was 'trying to put it down to imagination'. It was explained that the things he was experiencing were very real and perhaps frightening to him but that other people were not experiencing them.

There were still difficulties with John's hostile reactions to some patients and staff whom he did not like and who he threatened to 'stab' or 'get'. His reasons for this reaction were interesting and perhaps hold lessons for all nurses. 'The nurses speak to you as if you were a child, I know that I am younger than some people here but they speak as if I was a little girl . . . they just can't do that. People don't respect you . . . if you do everything a nurse tells you you get no respect, you become institutionalised and they trample all over you.'

Over a number of conversations it became clear

to me that John, even when well, would still resort to violence in order to assert himself if he felt others were taking advantage of him, whether male or female. He was finding it difficult to deal with the petty frustrations of hospital life. In the main nurses avoided violence by negotiating, explaining and reasoning but John could still bear a grudge for the slightest thing. Patients who had not developed these skills so keenly more often got into fights. For example, he punched David for 'invading my body space'. He later explained David had bumped into him and had 'just pushed his luck too far'. John did not accept that others might be ill and less skilled than himself so that when they behaved strangely he would dislike them and then bear a grudge. Nurses had to act as educators in putting other patients' behaviour in context.

Evaluation

Over the period of admission John was involved in seven violent incidents. Four involved assaults on other patients, once he was punched in the face, and he also smashed a chair and kicked at a door. He made a number of threats to nurses and other patients. During the attacks no one received serious injury, calm was quickly restored without the need for physical restraint or medication. These attacks were the result of disagreements and of John 'asserting' himself, except for smashing the chair which was displaced aggression.

In the latter part of his stay John was not violent. This he accounted for by saying 'If you're violent to other people then it makes life difficult for you, like you can't use the building in case there's someone waiting to take revenge'. I doubt from this statement that any long-term change has occurred and that should violence seem expedient in future it would be used.

Peplau's model has focused nursing attention on the 'why' of violence in attempting to understand the motivation and reasoning behind a violent action from the patient's viewpoint rather than imposing restrictions and force in order to suppress anger or violence. The following two examples illustrate this.

Situation 1

John got up from his chair and as he left the room kicked another patient. A nurse present says 'Hey, stop that, that's not done here'. John leaves the room.

Understanding

The nurse affirms that kicking is undesirable but does not know why it happened. John is aware that nurses disapprove of kicking.

Situation 2

John asks to borrow some money but is told it is not possible. He becomes threatening and abusive. When he is calm a nurse asks him to return to ask again and to listen to the reasons why it may not be possible. This he does.

Understanding

John is aggressive when his needs are not met. The nurse structures a situation to allow him to try to sort out new ways of dealing with the problem. He also gains reasons as to why it is not possible to borrow. He tests reality rather than feels 'got at' or 'tormented'.

Teaching John to live with needs that were not met immediately was a constant part of his nursing care. It is uncertain whether he was more able to defer his needs but it is certain that he no longer became violent when they were not met.

Peplau's model aids the nurse in her understanding of her role in the development of a relationship from admission through to discharge. It ensures that the nurse attempts to understand the experience of hospitalisation from the patient's viewpoint. There is, however, a danger of the nurse 'going native' and over-identifying with the patient, particularly as patients are primarily concerned with their own needs and perceptions while the nurse has to manage the needs of a group of people. I experienced particular difficulty in this and was aware that I was sometimes out of step with the views of my nursing colleagues.

Although the model directs nurses in the identification of problems, and to an extent in the formation of relationships, it does not explain how she is to fulfil her role as an educator. Any curriculum based on Peplau's model would require teaching on developmental psychology, counselling skills, psychotherapy, time for personal growth through supervision and analysis of oneself in relation to one's work, the management of change and a myriad other interpersonal skills (Peplau herself gives a comprehensive list).

The use of this model in a secure unit highlights other issues that were not resolved by reference to Peplau's original work. The 1983 Mental Health Act allows patients to be treated against their will if they are not able to consent or if a second opinion doctor agrees that the treatment is necessary in order to alleviate or prevent a deterioration of the patient's condition (Part 4, Section 58b). In such circumstances, help in the form of nursing and medical intervention may be seen by the patient as being coercive. The idea that the patient seeks help, as in the orientation phase, becomes redundant and unless the patient does eventually recognise that they need help they never enter the stages of a helping relationship that Peplau describes.

One particular aspect of patient care that this model assisted in was the reorientation John went through from being a prisoner in a hospital wing to a patient in a secure unit. This was evident from his first comment, when he said he had expected the hospital to be open. This work took a number of weeks and focused on John's ability and willingness to accept a need for help and his relationship with the nurses. At first John expected nurses to be like prison officers and was suspicious of their overtures to befriend him. Over a period of time he became more relaxed in these interactions and was made aware of what nurses and other staff could offer him both inside and outside of the hospital. This aspect of our work is often neglected and ex-prisoners regard themselves as 'doing time', and so never fully address their need to work on problems.

It is clear that as nurses begin to identify models of practice they are going to have to challenge the dominant medical model. For example, a mutually agreed need that centres on the troubling nature of auditory hallucinations may bring about the prescription of medication regardless of the patient or nurse's wish for other interventions. Help may be sought but the method of delivery may be usurped by the responsible medical officer. In terms of the power structure of psychiatry, the nurse and the patient may have little option but to comply. The question of whether a nurse can ever be an effective agent of change in the psychiatric setting remains unanswered. While the medical model dominates with its emphasis on physical treatments and the suppression of symptoms, the therapeutic possibilities of the nurse–patient relationship may never be more than an interesting sideline.

Nurses, too, have to work out whether they actually want to be involved in the business of helping people to look at their problems and learn to live with them, or whether they want a quiet life and a quiet ward. It may be that, while nursing continues to happen in institutions with their rules and regulations and the social pressure to maintain the status quo, Peplau's (or any nursing) model cannot be used to any great effect. For me, there is an inherent conflict between the nurse as 'keeper of the peace' and nurse as 'facilitator of change'.

It may be that before we consider which model of nursing best suits our needs or the needs of our clients we have to sort out our position within the multidisciplinary team. It is difficult to imagine two models working harmoniously side-by-side. They do not at present and while nurses work alongside other professionals they cannot simply go it alone.

References

Altschul A 1972 *Nurse–Patient Interaction.* Churchill Livingstone, Edinburgh.

Baldwin S 1983 Nursing models in special hospital settings. *Journal of Advanced Nursing*, 8: 473–476.

Barton R 1959 *Institutional Neurosis.* John Wright, Bristol.

Bell GM 1955 Provisions in the Mental Health Service. *British Medical Journal*, 1: 462–465.

Brown JS, Wooldridge PJ & van Bruggen Y 1973 Interpersonal relationships amongst psychiatric patients – the determinants of social attraction. *Journal of Health and Social Behaviour*, 14: 51–60.

Campbell W & Mawson D 1978 Violence in a psychiatric unit. *Journal of Advanced Nursing*, 3: 55–64.

Clack J 1963 Nursing intervention into the aggressive behaviour of patients. In *Some Clinical Approaches to Psychiatric Nursing*, SF Burd & MA Marshall (Eds). Macmillan, New York.

Cobb JP & Gossop MR 1976 Locked doors in the management of disturbed psychiatric patients. *Journal of Advanced Nursing*, 1: 469–480.

Cormack D 1973 *Psychiatric Nursing Observed.* RCN, London.

Dabbs JM 1971 Physical closeness and negative feelings. *Psychonomic Science*, 23: 141–143.

DHSS 1976 *Report of the Committee on Mentally Abnormal Offenders* (Butler Report). HMSO, London.

Doherty EG 1971 Social attraction and choice among psychiatric patients and staff: A review. *Journal of Health and Social Behaviour*, 12: 279–290.

Drinkwater J 1982 Violence in psychiatric hospitals. In *Developments in the Study of Criminal Behaviour*, P Feldman (Ed). John Wiley & Sons, Chichester.

Duggan S & Rix G 1987 A case study of communication. *Focus* (newsletter of Psychiatric Nurses Association), March 1987.

Emiley SF 1975 The effects of crowding and interpersonal attraction on affective responses, task performance and verbal behaviour. *The Journal of Social Psychology*, 97: 267–278.

Fottrell E 1980 A study of violent behaviour among patients in psychiatric hospitals. *British Journal of Psychiatry*, 136: 216–221.

Goffman I 1961 *Asylums.* Penguin, London.

Hodgkinson P, Hillis T & Russell D 1984 Assaults on staff in a psychiatric hospital. *Nursing Times*, 84, 15: 44–46.

Lee A 1980 A philosophy of care for the disturbed violent patient in a special hospital. *Nursing Times*, 76, 47: 2048–2051.

Lemmer B 1979 A slap in the face. *Nursing Mirror*, 149, 9: 18–19.

Mandlebrote B 1958 An experiment in the rapid conversion of a closed mental hospital into an open door hospital. *Mental Hygiene*, 42: 3–16.

Mental Health Act 1983 HMSO, London.

Menzies I 1960 *The Functioning of Social Systems as a Defence Against Anxiety.* Tavistock Publications, London.

Paulus P, Cox V, McCain G & Chandler J 1975 The effects of crowding in a prison environment. *Journal of Applied Psychology*, 5: 86–91.

Peplau HE 1952 *Interpersonal Relations in Nursing.* GP Putnam's Sons, New York.

Rogers CR 1961 *On Becoming a Person.* Constable & Co, London.

Salvage J 1985 *The Politics of Nursing.* Heinemann Medical, London.

Sommer R 1969 *Personal Space: The Behavioural Analysis of Design.* Prentice-Hall, Englewood Cliffs, New Jersey.

Taylor PJ 1982 Schizophrenia and violence. In *Abnormal Offenders, Delinquency and the Criminal Justice System*, J Gunn & DP Farrington (Eds). John Wiley & Sons, Chichester.

Taylor PJ (Unpub) Violence and psychosis: Three themes in a relationship. Cited in *Mental Illness, Personality Disorder and Offending: Issues of treatment and rehabilitation*, R Tullock, M McCulloch & R Fitzpatrick. Headley Bros, Kent.

Taylor PJ 1985 Motives for offending among violent and psychotic men. *British Journal of Psychiatry*, 147: 491–498.

Towell D 1975 *Understanding Psychiatric Nursing.* Royal College of Nursing, London.

Weaver SM, Armstrong NE, Broome AK & Stewart L 1978 Behavioural principles applied to a security ward. *Nursing Times*, 74, 1: 22–24.

Weaver SM, Broome AK & Kat BJB 1978 Some patterns of disturbed behaviour in a closed ward environment. *Journal of Advanced Nursing*, 3: 251–263.

11

Care plan for a suicidal person, using Roy's Adaptation model

Ian Moore

This chapter describes the use of the Roy Adaptation model in the care of a man believed to be at risk of committing suicide. The problem and incidence of suicide is discussed, and the nursing management of the suicidal patient is examined. Roy's (1970) Adaptation model is then described and a primary and secondary assessment, together with a care plan, are documented and discussed.

Suicide

Suicide is defined by Waltzer (1971) as a successfully fatal act of self injury, which an individual consciously undertakes.

Suicide is seen to be an intensely personal action but the underlying reasons for it are quite often found in the social relationships and interactions of the individual concerned. It is therefore not possible to understand the individual who commits suicide in isolation from his social background.

Statistics relating to suicide are often inaccurate. This may be due to difficulties in actually differentiating between a suicidal act and a fatal accident and, in addition, Kessel (1965) makes the suggestion that coroners are sometimes reluctant to

pass a verdict of suicide since this is regarded by many as a disgrace for the deceased.

Table 11.1 shows the suicide rates for England and Wales 1974 to 1984.

Table 11.2 shows the Registrar General's classification of suicidal acts and Table 11.3 shows male and female suicide rates from 1974 to 1984 according to this classification.

By reference to Tables 11.1 and 11.3 it can be observed that there are differences in the means by which men and women commit suicide. It is likely that these are, at least in part, due to the different socialisation of the sexes.

There appears to be a relationship between aggression and suicide, and West (1965) notes that one in three murderers commit suicide.

Freud (1920) suggests the idea of a death instinct, which he termed 'Thanatos'. The goal of this instinct is to achieve a complete and unalterable state of rest. The death instinct causes the individual to ignore new stimuli, and to return to earlier states of relative security at times of stress. It may be seen as a biological tendency to self-destruction, and the responses which it brings about in the person may be seen as maladaptive. Ordinarily, the instinct is rigorously controlled but

Table 11.1   Suicides in England and Wales, 1974–1984 (OPCS)

Year	1974	1975	1976	1977	1978	1979	1980	1981	1982	1983	1984
Male	2280	2184	2330	2363	2436	2564	2629	2761	2781	2812	2859
Female	1619	1509	1486	1581	1586	1631	1692	1658	1498	1467	1456
Total	3899	3693	3816	3944	4022	4195	4321	4419	4279	4279	4315

Table 11.2 Registrar General's classification of suicide (OPCS)

E950	Poisoning by solid or liquid substances
E951	Poisoning by gases in domestic use
E952	Poisoning by other causes
E953	By hanging, strangulation and suffocation
E954	By submersion (drowning)
E955	By fire arms and explosives
E956	By cutting and piercing instruments
E957	By jumping from high place
E958	By other and unspecified means
E959	Late effect of self-inflicted injury

is continuously trying to sever the connections with the outside world, which is the source of disturbing stimuli. If the ability to control this instinct is lost then the individual may withdraw from reality by retreating into a fantasy world or, in the extreme, by killing themselves.

Only in approximately one third of successful suicides is there an established psychiatric disorder. However, many more have consulted their general practitioner before the suicide. Waltzer (1971), in a study of a group of suicides, found that 65% had consulted their GP within the 3 to 4 months prior to the suicide occurring.

There are undoubtedly 'risk' factors which increase the likelihood of a person committing suicide. The following factors are associated with suicidal potential. Their presence indicates a suicidal risk and, on the admission of a client to hospital, they should be closely and carefully considered by the nurse carrying out an assessment.

Marital status The suicide rate for single people (including divorced, separated and widowed individuals) is greater than that of married people.

Sex Generally, more men than women commit suicide. It is suggested that biosocial influences may account, at least in part, for these differences. Grove and Tudor (1973), in a discussion of several studies of differential rates of mental illness, conclude that women experience more stress in marriage than men but that single men are more stressed than single women. Further, men are socialised into responding to frustration and stress in an aggressive way, and in a suicidal act this aggression is directed inwards onto the self. Men also appear likely to choose methods with a high chance of success, including hanging, shooting and

Table 11.3 Completed suicide by classification, 1974–1984: female (male). All age groups are included. (OPCS)

Year	1974	1975	1976	1977	1978	1979	1980	1981	1982	1983	1984
E950	(794) 1083	(709) 969	(684) 916	(675) 988	(680) 939	(709) 911	(653) 919	(647) 872	(576) 797	(589) 711	(495) 678
E951	(34) 16	(19) 4	(10) 4	(7) 1	(10) 1	(5) 4	(10)	(11) 1	(2) 2	(3)	(10) 1
E952	(275) 26	(249) 27	(306) 39	(433) 43	(363) 38	(419) 52	(436) 46	(564) 64	(649) 66	(585) 81	(773) 90
E953	(579) 182	(593) 220	(698) 256	(631) 237	(694) 273	(711) 283	(770) 291	(790) 330	(830) 289	(881) 340	(891) 326
E954	(129) 161	(140) 144	(115) 141	(141) 141	(133) 138	(142) 166	(142) 205	(153) 177	(115) 151	(133) 116	(92) 141
E955	(154) 8	(143) 17	(171) 6	(146) 10	(180) 9	(175) 12	(212) 7	(179) 8	(165) 13	(207) 13	(205) 12
E956	(76) 21	(59) 20	(72) 18	(72) 27	(86) 22	(93) 27	(72) 30	(79) 24	(81) 25	(89) 20	(77) 23
E957	(100) 55	(110) 46	(106) 43	(87) 67	(98) 83	(116) 85	(112) 83	(79) 47	(81) 38	(119) 81	(114) 77
E958	(139) 67	(162) 62	(167) 63	(171) 67	(192) 83	(193) 91	(222) 111	(259) 135	(282) 117	(206) 105	(202) 108
E959			(1)			(1)					

jumping. This is in contrast to methods such as wrist-cutting and taking an overdose of tranquillisers (Hoff, 1978).

Loss   The loss of a close personal relationship through bereavement or separation may bring about a suicide. In addition, the *threat* of loss (whether real or imagined), including loss of status or job, may precipitate such a response.

Age   The elderly are more likely to commit suicide than any other age group. This is partly due to the increased probability of the occurrence of one or more of the other factors, the most significant of these being loss.

Previous attempts or gestures regardless of the intent. The individual may be trying to gain attention but even a slight miscalculation in the dosage of drugs or the mistiming of a telephone call for help, will result in a successful suicide. The risk is increased if the individual has made a previous attempt that would have been successful if treatment had not been received. It would appear that the more violent and painful the attempt, the greater the risk of success at the next attempt.

Alcohol and drug abuse   There is a prevalence of substance abuse in most age groups. Alcohol and drugs can blunt inhibitions about suicide and reduce the pain involved in an attempt. Withdrawal of alcohol and drugs may also increase the risk of suicide due to the state of unease, discomfort and distress.

Depression   Suicidal risk is increased when there is a history of depressive illness. This risk is exacerbated by drug and alcohol abuse.

Hallucinatory states   These significantly increase the risk, particularly when the person is taunted by merciless voices which may instruct him to kill himself.

Religion   Active participation within any religion appears to be associated with lower than average suicide rates. In part, this may be explained by the belief that taking life is 'against God's will'. However, this lower incidence is also encountered among members of those faiths which condone suicide. Religious faith may bring with it a sense of order and stability, and the suffering experienced in

life may be seen as the price to be paid for everlasting salvation and hence be more bearable.

University students show an increased suicide rate. The results of a study by Lyman (1961) of student suicides, reported the suicide rates in the 20–24 age group shown in Table 11.4.

Table 11.4   Suicide rates in 1961, per 1 000 000 population, at Oxford, Cambridge, London and seven unnamed universities (Lyman, 1961)

Oxford University	26.4
Cambridge University	21.3
University of London	16.3
Seven unnamed universities	5.6
This age group in England and Wales	4.1

It would appear that university students are exposed to greater stress than their counterparts in the general population. In addition, Rook (1959) has suggested that the fact that a greater proportion of students at Oxford, Cambridge and in London live in halls of residence may account for the differences indicated in Table 11.4. This, he suggests, increases loneliness and introspection.

Occupation appears to be an important factor in suicide. Individuals who are employed in professional occupations have a higher suicide rate than skilled workers. The suicide rates for unskilled workers are also higher than those of skilled workers.

People suffering from *organic mental disorders* may be considered as being at risk, particularly people whose organic mental disorder fluctuates. When depression is associated with an organic mental syndrome, increased confusion may lessen the intensity of the depressive symptoms and a corresponding decrease in suicidal impulses. However, as the confusion lessens, the depressive symptoms will often recur and may precipitate a suicidal attempt.

Individuals with poor mechanisms of personal and social adaptation are also at greater risk; particularly when these are associated with isolation, loneliness and an inability to cope.

Suicide rates indicate a *seasonal variation*. The period that most suicides occur appears to be late spring and early summer, with another peak in the autumn. As yet there is no satisfactory explanation for this.

A *family history* of suicide does increase the risk of other family members committing suicide and, since there is no evidence that an inherited depressive tendency is responsible, it is likely that stigma and social isolation are important factors in explaining this increased risk.

Although the specific aetiology of suicidal acts remains vague, a person is more likely to commit a suicidal act if his life-situation includes any of the suicide risk factors outlined. Obviously, the more of these risk factors which are present, the greater is the risk of a successful suicide.

Therefore, assessment and evaluation of suicide risk factors should be an urgent and integral part of any admission and evaluation procedure.

Nursing the suicidal patient

The nursing care and management of patients who are actively suicidal may be trying and difficult, and bring into play the moral and social dilemmas of human rights and the sanctity of life. Nurses, traditionally, have been concerned with the preservation of life. This concern has been used to justify interventions in physical illness and, for example, the use of restraint in coping with the emotionally disturbed. However, as Szasz (1974) suggests, the freedom to choose the time and place of one's death may be viewed as a basic human right, whatever the preferred method (hanging or drowning, smoking or alcohol abuse). Self-examination on the part of the nurse is therefore necessary, in order to decide one's own standpoint and to decide *if*, and if so *when*, coercive intervention is justifiable.

Within psychiatric hospitals there are two main methods of attempting to prevent suicide.

1 *A controlled environment* The area in which the patient is cared for is rigorously controlled to exclude as many objects as possible which could be used in a suicide attempt.
2 *Continuous observation* A member of the nursing staff is with the patient continuously throughout the day and night, until the risk is considered to have abated.

Neither of these methods of managing a suicidal patient is entirely satisfactory because:

(a) A ward environment is created which can offer encouragement to patients who are not suicidal, but who are attention-seeking, to indulge in suicidal gestures.
(b) A patient who is actively suicidal may not display any suicidal behaviour whilst he is aware of obvious monitoring.
(c) Some suicidal patients may feel that they must pit their wits against the system of monitoring and supervision, and overcome it.

In practice, one or a mixture of both of these methods is generally applied. As far as can be determined, this is due to a now very serious fear that accusations of negligence and litigation would follow in the event of a successful suicide attempt. More realistic methods of management involve the use of single-storey psychiatric units, and a ward design which will permit good observation throughout the ward so that observation of individual patients can be unobtrusive.

Only one consultant psychiatrist should be responsible for any one ward. Different consultants have differing requirements, which may create areas of conflict among both medical and nursing staff.

Adequate staffing ratios may avoid unnecessary stress being placed on staff, and may even reduce staff sickness/absence figures.

Continuity of medical and nursing staff is essential to avoid disruption and instability.

The attitudes of staff play an important part, though it is difficult to measure. As a general observation, suicide attempts appear to decline when the staff appear calm and unworried, and to increase when the staff appear anxious under stress.

The Roy Adaptation model

The Roy (1970) Adaptation model of nursing is particularly suitable for use in psychiatric care. The model seeks to examine the following:

1   The essential qualities of the client who is to receive nursing care.
2   The aetiology of the client's problems which may need nursing intervention.
3   The nursing assessment of the client.
4   The planning of nursing care and the construction of client-related goals.
5   The type of nursing intervention necessary during the implementation of nursing care.
6   The evaluation of the quality and effects of the nursing care given.

Roy (1970) acknowledges that the Adaptation model owes much to the work of Harry Helson, a psychologist who developed a psychological theory of adaptation.

Helson (1964) states that physiological and psychological systems exist in conditions of relative stability, which the person will try to maintain. This stability is the best that the person can achieve for himself. However, there is no absolutely correct balance, but there exists a broad range of responses through which the person will function and cope with an ever-changing environment. Clients may be seen as attempting to maintain their physiological, self-conception, role function and interdependency systems within an environment which is unique to them.

Roy (1970) states that the client's internal and external environments make up the client's adaptation level. Accordingly, new stimuli which are within the existing adaptation level will achieve a more positive reaction than those which are outside it.

According to Roy, three types of stimuli are the factors which will determine the client's adaptation level at any given moment. These stimuli are called:

1   *Focal stimuli* These are the stimuli which immediately confront the client.
2   *Contextual stimuli* These are all the other stimuli which are present.
3   *Residual stimuli* These are factors from past experiences which may be relevant to the current situation but whose effects cannot be validated. They include attitudes and beliefs.

Clients may be viewed as comprising four subsystems. These subsystems influence behaviour

and are termed 'modes of adaptation', and consist of:

1   The *physiological* mode of adaptation. This covers a very wide range of activity. The ability of a client to cope successfully with new stimuli is related to the nature of the stimuli themselves and to the client's current mode of physiological adaptation.
2   The *self-concept* mode of adaptation. This is an extremely complex mode and is determined by the view which the person holds of himself through his interaction with others.
3   The *role-function* mode of adaptation. This relates to the client carrying out a set of duties within given roles. However, this may create a sense of failure, or even conflict, when the client's ability to carry out the duties of the assumed roles is beyond the range to which he can successfully adapt.
4   The *interdependence* mode of adaptation. This is particularly affected by the client's internal and external environments. It involves the client's methods of seeking and dealing with such interpersonal relationships, including love, hostility, attention, friendship, dominance and aggression.

The four modes of adaptation have been represented in the form of a diagram in Fig. 11.1. The planning and delivery of nursing care focuses on the ability of the client's modes of adaptation to cope with varying degrees of success with the stimuli.

Thus, according to Roy, nursing activity is aimed at assisting the client's adaptation to his physiological, self-concept role-function and interdependency modes in both sickness and health.

Using the Roy Adaptation model together with the nursing process, the stages of patient care can be represented schematically (Fig. 11.2).

The nursing assessment

This is divided into two parts: primary and secondary assessment.

Fig. 11.1 The four modes of adaptation (Roy 1970)

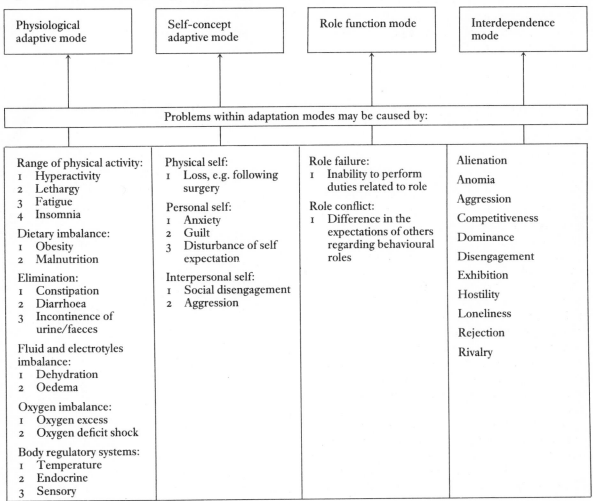

Physiological adaptive mode	Self-concept adaptive mode	Role function mode	Interdependence mode

Problems within adaptation modes may be caused by:

Range of physical activity: 1 Hyperactivity 2 Lethargy 3 Fatigue 4 Insomnia Dietary imbalance: 1 Obesity 2 Malnutrition Elimination: 1 Constipation 2 Diarrhoea 3 Incontinence of urine/faeces Fluid and electrotyles imbalance: 1 Dehydration 2 Oedema Oxygen imbalance: 1 Oxygen excess 2 Oxygen deficit shock Body regulatory systems: 1 Temperature 2 Endocrine 3 Sensory	Physical self: 1 Loss, e.g. following surgery Personal self: 1 Anxiety 2 Guilt 3 Disturbance of self expectation Interpersonal self: 1 Social disengagement 2 Aggression	Role failure: 1 Inability to perform duties related to role Role conflict: 1 Difference in the expectations of others regarding behavioural roles	Alienation Anomia Aggression Competitiveness Dominance Disengagement Exhibition Hostility Loneliness Rejection Rivalry

Primary assessment

This must be carried out accurately. The client's behaviour in each mode of adaptation is observed and carefully examined in turn, and those modes within which there exists adaptation problems are identified. Naturally, should there be no adaptation problems in any of the modes, then the assessment can be terminated at this point as there is no need for nursing intervention.

Secondary assessment

This involves the identification of the specific focal, contextual and residual stimuli which are respons-

ible for the adaptation problems which have been identified. It is Roy's contention that the factors which determine the client's ability to adapt may be considered as focal, contextual and residual stimuli. These stimuli, with their relationship to a client's adaptation level, will cause the client to behave in the manner he does. There is a need to examine the extent to which each of these types of stimuli may be considered as affecting the client's behaviour.

Other factors are also involved in the nursing assessment and will affect the identification of the modes of adaptation which are manifesting adapta-

Fig. 11.2 Schematic view of the Roy Adaptation model. Evaluation is seen as a continuous process

SUICIDE

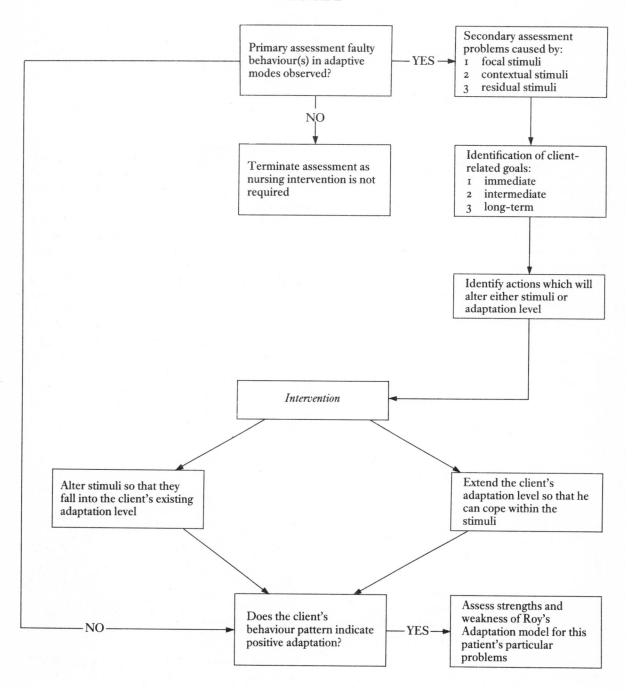

tion problems and the identification of the specific stimuli involved. These are

1 the quality and nature of the nurse–client relationship, and
2 the extent to which the client has an active role in the assessment process.

Planning and goal setting

With the information gathered from the nursing assessment, a list of client-related goals is drawn up, specifying what the client ought to be able to do when the goal is achieved. These goals are then placed in an order of priority and are divided into immediate, intermediate and long-term units of achievement.

Short-term goals will usually involve extending the client's adaptation level, within one or more modes of adaptation.

Intermediate goals often involve extending the client's adaptation level and changing appropriate stimuli.

Long-term goals involve helping the client to adapt positively and effectively with an environment that is always changing.

Nursing intervention

This involves the manipulation of the relationship between the environmental stimuli and the client's adaptation level. The effect of the manipulation is to allow stimuli to fall within the client's adaptation zone. This may be achieved by either selection of stimuli to fall within the client's current range of adaptation, or the rejection of those stimuli that are outside the client's adaptation zone. Potentially, there are three ways of doing this:

(a) active – the nurse selects the stimuli for the client;
(b) passive – the client's environment is used to filter and select appropriate stimuli;
(c) manipulation of the client's present adaptation level.

The Roy Model of Adaptation implies that each client is attempting to achieve a state of relative physiological and psychological balance. Therefore, the aim of nursing intervention is to effect a change in the adaptation level to enable the client to cope with the stimuli.

Initially, the focal stimuli will be the subject of manipulation as they are the primary cause of the client's behaviour, and then consideration is given to extending the adaptation zone.

Nursing evaluation

If this is to be accurate and successful then the goals must be set during the planning stage of the nursing process. These goals are client-related and indicate the client's expected behaviour pattern following successful nursing intervention.

Therefore, when using the Roy Adaptation model in the planning of care, the behaviour in the effected adaptive mode is identified (physiological, role function, self-conception and interdependency). By the use of continuous evaluation throughout the delivery of care and the comparison of actual and predicted client behaviour patterns, the progress toward the units of achievement may be measured. Successful nursing intervention does not always occur. In this event, reassessment must take place and the process of planning and intervention is repeated or changed until nursing intervention is successful. This process is shown schematically in Fig. 11.2.

Client history

Mr John Lay, aged 66, was born in Canton, China. From the age of 11 he attended a boarding school, where he was very unhappy. After failing his Oxford entrance examinations, he enlisted in the Royal Navy at the outbreak of World War II, and was based at a shore establishment. In 1941, after a short engagement, he was married. By October 1942 John had become very anxious and overactive and this led to his being hospitalised in Portsmouth and receiving a medical discharge in January 1943.

In March 1945 John obtained employment as a junior manager. He proved to be a capable employee and gained promotion.

By January 1952 it became obvious that his father was dying of cancer and, as the months passed, John became increasingly solitary, introverted and morbid. On the death of his father in December 1952, John had become deeply depressed. After seeing a psychiatrist, he was admitted to hospital in February 1953 with a diagnosis of depression. He received a course of 10 modified electro-convulsive therapy sessions, and in June 1953 was discharged.

During September 1968 his mother died of bronchopneumonia. This appeared to unsettle John and he became both physically and mentally overactive. By the end of September 1968 he was in a hypomanic state and was admitted to a psychiatric hospital. Treatment consisted of lithium carbonate 2G daily and chlorpromazine 100 mg four times daily and he was discharged in November 1968.

For the next 18 years John lived in the community. This period was not an easy one, and was marked by John's variation in mood. He also developed an interest in politics and periodically attended the local meetings of a political party. Politics tended to become a barometer of John's mood. When he was feeling 'on top of the world', he acknowledged only one viewpoint, his own, and no matter how irrational this was he would try to impress it upon others, particularly at political meetings! In addition, he would write to the Prime Minister of the time and insist that he, and not the Prime Minister, represented the party. When feeling low, he would seclude himself, sometimes for days, and bemoan the fate and politics of the nation. At times, he would threaten his wife; on one occasion he physically attacked her. The marital relationship became very strained and eventually his wife commenced divorce proceedings.

The divorce was finalised in July 1986 and John became depressed. After initial treatment by his general practitioner, he was referred for a psychiatric opinion. After being interviewed by the psychiatrist, John was admitted in September 1986.

Fig. 11.3 Primary assessment

Name: John Lay	Date of birth: 31.03.20
Date of admission: 06.09.86	Age: 66
Mental health status: Informal	Marital status: Divorced

General information: Divorced 2 months ago. On admission, was untidily dressed. Poor standard of personal hygiene. Appears depressed. Little response to happenings on the ward. Sits very still. Movements appear to be very slow. Poor concentration. Speech is monotonous.

Maladaptive behaviour in following modes:

Physiological	Self-concept	Role function	Interdependence
Loss of appetite	Low self-esteem	Dissatisfied with life	Feels isolated
Easily fatigued	Pessimistic about his future	Not interested in former	Does not feel to be a part
Sleep disturbance –	Doubts value of his life	pastimes	of society
wakes up early	Feels guilty and remorseful	Feels helpless	Feels lonely
Constipated	about his ill-treatment of	Wishes to cry but cannot	Little motivation
	his wife	Feels that he has failed in	
	Poor concentration	life	
	No obvious suicidal	Feels hopeless	
	thoughts		
	No obvious delusions or		
	hallucinations		

Summary: Maladaptive behaviours found in all four modes of adaptation. No overt signs of suicidal behaviour, but appears very depressed. Intervention required. Refer to secondary assessment.

Fig. 11.4 Secondary assessment

Focal stimuli	Contextual stimuli	Residual stimuli
Recent divorce.	The ward environment is providing the bulk of the contextual stimuli. Currently, the ward situation is very tense, due to the provocative behaviour of Mrs G, who is attempting to gain the attention of staff and fellow patients by making suicide attempts and gestures. The medical and nursing staff appear tense and anxious. Visitors appear to be very concerned about Mrs G. The concern is being expressed to the nursing staff. Concern regarding Mrs G. is also being expressed by her fellow patients. However, they appear somewhat more philosophical about the situation.	John's past experiences of depressive illness, his attitudes, traits and other past learning experiences are contributing to his feelings of hopelessness. John has expressed the idea that he wonders how long he can go on. However, he does acknowledge that his depression will lift, although he does believe that it is more or less inevitable that the depression will return.

Fig. 11.5 Care plan

Problem	Goal	Intervention	Evaluation
Potential suicide.	John will not harm himself.	Observe for evidence of suicidal intent. Accompany when leaving ward.	
Depressed thoughts and feelings evident in conversation.	Depressive rumination will diminish.	One-to-one discussion twice a day. Explain physical effects of depression. Commence antidepressant medication. Occupational therapy-basic craft. Assess concentration and motivation.	8.9.86 More animated. Relating to Staff Nurse D. 9.9.86 Quiet and isolated.
Diminished appetite. Constipated.	Re-establish usual food and fluid (2.5 l/day) intake. Re-establish normal bowel habit (every other day).	Give dietary supplements and extra drinks 150 ml/hour	7.9.86 Food intake poor. Fluid intake satisfactory.
Isolated, not mixing on ward.	Gradual socialisation, expression of individuality. Regain social skills.	Accompany to group activities: open discussion group and art therapy. Discuss with John and identify deficits.	7.9.86 Quiet and isolated.
Sleep disturbance: early morning wakening.	Sleep for 6 hours each night.	Monitor sleep pattern: sleep chart. Night sedation if required.	

Fig. 11.6   Excerpts from John's day

7.9.86

Quiet and isolated. John appears very concerned over the behaviour of Mrs G, who is making suicidal gestures. Please nurse these two people in different ward areas. Diet remains poor, fluid intake satisfactory.

8.9.86

John appears more animated today. Becoming agitated?
At 17.30 hours Mrs G absconded from the ward. John is very concerned about her and has offered to help search for her with nursing staff. At approximately 19.30 hours Mrs G was returned to the ward by the police. She appears to be seeking and getting John's attention.
John appears to be relating well with Staff Nurse D, who is concerned that he identifies with Mrs G and her problems.

9.9.86

Appears very quiet and isolated. Not communicating with anyone. Please observe.
At 19.30 hours, John found to be missing. Last positively seen at 19.20 hours, in television lounge. Has not been observed near the ward doors. Therefore, it is likely that he left the ward by a window. The hospital ground search was implemented at 19.35 hours. Medical staff, next of kin, police and administration informed at 19.40 hours.
22.00 hours, telephone message from police. They have recovered a body from a local river. The general description is that of John.
22.30 hours, nursing staff positively identify body as that of John Lay.

Evaluation

During both the primary and secondary stages of John's admission assessment (Figs 11.3 and 11.4) no overt signs of suicidal behaviour were detected. However, John was deemed to be a potential suicide risk because there was an obvious depressive illness present and because there were present other factors indicating suicide risk. The way in which these were documented is discussed later in this section.

It must be noted that the determination of the suicidal patient to achieve his objective should never be underestimated. Unless this determination can be channelled into more constructive areas then the prognosis must be ultimately very poor despite any preventative measures that may have been taken.

There is an assumption commonly made by the general public, nursing staff, medical staff and the media that a suicide occurring within a psychiatric hospital is related to negligence or to unprofessionalism. This assumption is grossly unfair. Despite adequate precautions and the awareness of a potential suicide risk, there is a very real possibility that the staff will be unable to prevent a successful suicide attempt. A suicide brings tragedy, bitterness and misery to family, friends and the medical and nursing staff involved. Quite often, the family and friends will believe that it could have been prevented. Usually, this will produce bitterness and feelings of recrimination that may be expressed by complaints about individual members of staff and the threat of litigation.

Within the Roy Adaptation model, the role of the nurse is to act as an external force, which regulates and modifies the stimuli which affect adaptation. By assuming this role the nurse must remember that she may become a focus for any feelings of bitterness and allegations of negligence that a relative or friend of the deceased may choose to make. Therefore, nursing staff must learn to cope in an effective manner with the aftermath of a successful suicide.

Firstly, it is necessary to examine the circumstances of the incident and to identify positive and negative aspects of nursing intervention. The purpose of this would not be to apportion blame, but to learn from the event so that action may be taken to remedy any errors of omission or commission or to carry forward any new insights to future, similar, situations. Secondly, the response of the friend or relative should not be reacted to in a defensive or dismissive way. Anger is a common reaction to loss, and may be a prominent feature of the grieving process. It should also be remembered that society is still largely conditioned by Judaeo-Christian ethics. These ethics are quite powerful and within them suicide is often equated with sin.

The model in practice

It could be suggested that the Roy Adaptation model helped to identify John as being at risk. In practice, the idea of focal and contextual stimuli served to draw attention to factors in John's background and current circumstances which corresponded with those discussed earlier in this chapter. In this way they were included in a more formal assessment framework than would otherwise have been the case. Generally, it appears that the recognition of such factors occurs at an intuitive level and tends to be idiosyncratic rather than coordinated.

In this instance, suicidal risk factors were identified during the first-stage assessment, and subsequently amongst the contextual and residual stimuli. It could be suggested that this kind of classification leads to such stimuli being regarded as a low priority simply because they are not 'focal'. This may have been the case with John in that all nurses may not have been convinced of the seriousness of the risk. For a unified response to occur, all nurses would need to be familiar with the elements of Roy's model and to understand the way in which problems are identified.

Another aspect highlighted by this care study is that factors such as the layout of the ward, which may or may not be significant with a particular patient, will nevertheless be taken into account as contextual stimuli. Thus, the model offers a new way of looking at the situation so that the interaction between the person and their environment becomes more significant. In this way, the environment would be examined in relation to each patient. In retrospect it appears that difficulties were experienced with adopting this perspective.

Difficulties were also identified in relation to the use of unfamiliar documentation, which manifested themselves in the framing and wording of patient problems. However, it is recognised that this latter criticism relates not so much to the use of this particular model in practice, but to attempts to introduce patient-centred care. If the use of a nursing model serves to bring alive the nursing process, then it may also serve to highlight deficiencies in the implementation of the nursing process.

Nevertheless, one possible solution may be to modify the documentation to emphasise appropriate contextual and residual stimuli, so that problems may be readily identified, progress monitored and evaluation facilitated.

Finally, for the model to achieve acceptance its utility in a variety of situations would have to be demonstrated, and this has not yet been done.

References

Freud S 1920 *The complete psychological works of Sigmund Freud.* James J Strachey (Ed). Hogarth Press, London.

Grove WR & Tudor JF 1973 Adult sex roles and mental illness. *American Journal of Sociology*, 78: 812–835.

Helson H 1964 *Adaptation Level Theory.* Harper & Row, New York.

Hoff LA 1978 *People in Crisis: Understanding and Helping.* Addison-Wesley, Menlo Park, California.

Kessel WIN 1965 Self-poisoning I and II. *British Medical Journal*, 2, 1265, 1336: 790–798.

Lyman JL 1961 Student suicide at Oxford University. *Student Medicine*, 10: 218.

Office of Population Censuses and Surveys *Mortality Statistics 1974–84.* HMSO, London.

Rook A 1959 Student suicides. *British Medical Journal*, 1: 599.

Roy C 1970 Adaptation: A conceptual framework for nursing. *Nuring Outlook*, 18, 3: 42.

Szasz T 1974 *The Second Skin.* Routledge & Kegan Paul, London.

Waltzer M 1971 The suicidal patient and the medical practitioner. *Modern Medicine*, 16, 7: 13–16.

West DJ 1965 *Murder Followed by Suicide.* Heinemann, London.

12
Postscript
Blair Collister

Psychiatric nurses are used to practising in settings where more than one model of treatment and care operates. This point, discussed elsewhere (Collister, 1986) is supported in two ways by the chapters in this book.

Firstly, the ease with which contributors entered into the spirit of this work suggests they are not discomfited by being asked to consider approaches which differ from their usual perspective. Secondly, the general tenor and specific points discussed in each chapter indicate an awareness of a multi-dimensional approach to care and treatment. In other words, psychiatric nurses are aware that there may be several opinions about a given situation and are used to taking these into account in their clinical practice. Indeed, it is obvious that some contributors have been employing a deliberative approach to nursing care and a particular model for some time, and their chapters represent concrete evidence of these efforts. It may also be that, for other contributors, the work for this book provided the impetus (and excuse) necessary to try out a nursing model for the first time instead of the biomedical model customarily employed, and thereby provided the opportunity for experimenting.

Each contributor has discussed points which are specific to the application of a particular model and, although it is not possible to make generalisations from the work documented here, it is possible to draw conclusions and to suggest implications.

Various writers, including Riehl and Roy (1980) and Fitzpatrick and Whall (1983) have classified nursing models according to the main theoretical principle on which each is based. Thus, models are placed into categories such as 'developmental', 'systems' and so on. Models are then analysed for their internal consistency in their use of terms, and for their external validity. Whilst this is a valid academic exercise, it does not serve to indicate the practical use of the models so analysed. It is suggested that this latter purpose is served by the kind of work undertaken for, and documented in, this book. As a consequence, one of the conclusions which may be suggested concerns the general type of model which may have practical value in psychiatric nursing. Work on editing each chapter and the overview which develops as a result of this work leads to the suggestion that it is possible to identify two general types of models of nursing.

A typology of nursing models

Of the two general types of nursing model identified, the first seeks to make sense of the person through the identification of discrete elements which go together to make up the individual. However, rather than focusing on the *going together*, the tendency seems to be to emphasise the *separation* of these elements and to reduce the person to a series of fragments. This type of model may therefore be termed *reductionist*, and models of this type include those based on systems theory and those which incorporate activities of living or their equivalent.

The other type of model tends to focus on the nurse–patient relationship. Whilst both types of model employ a planned approach to care embodying the nursing process, the difference between them lies in the process which is being addressed. Models which focus on the nurse–patient relationship have the process of evolution of that relationship as their theme, rather than the cyclical problem-solving process inherent in reductionist models.

One conclusion which may be drawn from the chapters in this book is that *reductionist* models tend to be less satisfactory than *non-reductionist* models. Dissatisfaction with reductionist models appears to arise from one or more of the following observations.

1   Despite the assertion of theorists that their model is holistic, experience reveals that nursing assessments and care plans tend to be fragmented. Problems are identified in isolation and care planned accordingly.

It is not until the care plan is put into operation that the nursing action reintegrates perception of the individual as a whole being and even this may depend on the knowledge and skill of the practitioner. This fragmentation extends to the process of nursing itself, where the steps (assessing, planning, giving and evaluating care) are seen as discrete and efforts are directed to completing one stage before embarking on the next.

2   It is claimed that the nursing process and the attendant use of a nursing model provide an individualised approach to nursing care. However, it appears that a mechanistic approach (inherent in a reductionist-type model) means that the goals and interventions are routinised rather than individualised. Thus the care as documented may appear to be no more than what is usually done, dressed up in the jargon of the model. Part of the reason for this lies in the way in which the nursing process and, latterly, nursing models have been thrust upon practitioners without adequate or appropriate preparation. Part of the answer lies in the points made towards the end of the introductory chapter to this book, when nurse teachers and managers were encouraged to approach the introduction of change in a constructive and deliberative way.

3   In some instances, significant aspects of patient care appear to be inadequately addressed by a model or, more seriously, missed altogether. Herein lies a paradox. The inadequacies of the models have been identified and described here by experienced practitioners who possess the knowledge and skill necessary to enable them to recognise these shortcomings. If the models were to be employed by inexperienced or disinterested nurses then the consequences might be grave, both for nurses and patients. A nursing model is not a substitute for good nursing care, and poor practice will not improve merely by the use of a nursing model. It is the attendant changes in nurse education and concern over the quality of practice which will improve care.

Using the non-reductionist models, care plans do include precise, measurable goals. However, although these goals give direction to each interaction they do not interfere with, or constrain the dynamics of that interaction. The 'means', in human terms, are of at least equal importance to the 'ends' of care. Thus the nurse can employ his or her skills in each encounter with a particular patient and although the overall goal will remain the same the uniqueness and individuality of both nurse and patient can manifest itself.

Values

This fundamental dichotomy between reductionist and non-reductionist models may be examined by taking account of the values implicit in general human conduct and experience, and in the use of a particular type of model.

Within a reductionist model the 'worth' of a patient may partly depend on judgements about the progress he is or is not making in relation to care plan goals. The esteem in which the patient is held by the nurse is conditional upon the patient maintaining goal-directed progress, and not slipping back. This is not a criticism of the contributors to this text, but of the models they have used. In a sense it reflects the kind of reaction which occurs when a patient, viewed from a biomedical perspective, fails to respond to treatment, develops complications or suffers a relapse. There is a sense of failure on the part of the staff which may be projected onto the patient.

An implicit assumption, therefore, is that if the nurse does what has been prescribed (planned) then the patient could, indeed should, respond as expected.

Non-reductionist models, on the other hand, do recognise that the patient as a person has an obligation to respond in a manner which will help him, assuming it is safe to do so. However, and more fundamentally, these models also recognise that this may not always be possible. Before goal-directed progress occurs, regression may take place. Further, they acknowledge that the nurse may experience negative emotions, rejection and frustration. The skills of the nurse lie in being able to recognise and cope with these emotions without experiencing a loss of self-esteem which may then be projected onto the patient. In this way the nurse and the patient together learn, develop and grow through the dynamics of their mutual understanding.

For this to occur, two preconditions exist. The first is that nurses should be aware of the kind of values which underpin reductionist and non-reductionist models, and the influence of these values on their perception of the patient. The second is that some sort of support system is necessary to enable the nurse to recognise and cope with the variety of emotions engendered by such nursing practice. Whichever type of model is used, conflicts will arise which will require counsel and support in their resolution.

The relationship of nursing to medicine

Within these chapters, the relationship between the doctor and the nurse appears to show the features of one of the following three scenarios.

The hierarchy

In this scenario, the doctor is at the head and makes all significant decisions. Conflict may occur if opinions differ as to what may be the best approach to take. This conflict can be avoided if, for example, nurses ignore the existence of the doctor or his instructions. This ploy is helped if the actions are 'invisible' in the sense that no evidence will exist whether or not they are carried out. Nevertheless a power play takes place with the patient as a pawn in the game. Often, other subordinate staff are relegated to the same level as the patient, communication is poor and decisions are made in the absence of those most directly affected.

These decisions are not only about patient care and patient allocation for example, but also about off-duty and staff transfer.

Autonomy

In this situation the nurse or nurses work independently, enjoying the freedom to make their own decisions. However, accountability and who holds it may not be clear unless an error of omission or commission occurs. Clear demarcation lines are required and in this way a nursing model can contribute to the discussion about what lies within the domain of nursing. However, this may also lead to disputes over power and about who has control of which part of the patient's life.

Multidisciplinary

This would appear to be the optimal scenario evident in these chapters. Each recognises the contribution, rights and obligations of the other professions involved. According to the situation and the skills of the participants, decisions are made and acted upon by the most appropriate team member. In dealing with a particular problem this key worker may seek help but does not relinquish 'control' of the situation which is shared with the patient/client. Of particular note in the context of the obligations of particular team members is the acceptance by others of specific legal and other requirements. Thus the responsibility of medical staff with regard to admissions and discharges is recognised without jealousy, as is the responsibility of nursing staff with regard to such matters as professional conduct, the administration of medication and the safety of staff and patients. From a legal and moral perspective the buck stops somewhere, and those with whom the ultimate responsibility lies have a right to expect the support of other team members in discharging that responsibility.

Aside from the interdisciplinary tensions and harmonies which have been described, another contrast between nursing and medicine has been highlighted in some chapters. This contrast centres on clinical practice.

The use of a nursing model has resulted in the patient being seen in a more holistic way, and not just as the recipient of physical treatment. As a consequence, additional significant factors in the patient's background and circumstances have been recognised and this has led to the identification of problems which might otherwise have been missed. These problems go beyond those which relate to the nurse's traditional role in relation to medicine, and their solution of necessity has been achieved without recourse to medical intervention. Thus unique approaches have been implemented with demonstrable success.

Such approaches may serve to establish and reinforce the parameters of nursing and to indicate the uniqueness of the nursing input as different from but complementary to psychiatric medicine. The purpose of this would not be to establish rivalry but to highlight the need for interdisciplinary cooperation in the care and treatment of patients.

Conclusion

This postscript has suggested that two general types of model may be identified and this implies that nursing models may be classified conveniently into one or other category. However, it is recognised that this is not the case and that a model which may have the general features of one of the two types which have been described, may not always operate as such. Thus a model which could be regarded as reductionist may display none of the shortcomings of these models when used in practice. In part this is likely to be due to the skills and knowledge of the practitioner who recognises and compensates for the inadequacies of the model. In addition it is likely that the general nature of nursing models is appreciated. Thus activities of living or self care requisites are seen not as parts of a patient, but as a convenient means of classifying knowledge and skills to facilitate the acquisition of these for practice. Once these skills and knowledge have been acquired, the activities or requisites are referred to merely as an *aide-mémoire* and not as a rigid structure. The nurse's interaction with the patient therefore transcends the categorisation of biological, psychological and social information and the classification of problems, to include the means of obtaining the information so categorised and the solution of problems so classified. What matters then is not in which box or column a problem is written, but the meaning of the problem to the patient and the best means of solving the problem through the medium of the nurse–patient relationship.

It has also been suggested that one type of model appears less satisfactory than the other type. It is emphasised that this is based on the implications of the work in this book alone, and this reflects the lack of empirical investigation into the appropriateness and utility of nursing models.

This chapter has also drawn attention to other significant implications of using nursing models. The values implicit in a particular nursing model must be recognised and understood, and they must be accepted if a model is to have utility. If they cannot be accepted then the model has no utility.

From a management perspective the way in which a model is implemented must reflect the principles of the model itself. Finally, from the point of view of nurse education it is necessary that a model is recognised for what it is. It is the understanding which the model offers, and the knowledge and skills which it implicates and explicates which are the substance of nursing practice, and hence the curriculum.

In another context, Goffman (1961) has suggested that the institution not only defines the member as a member but also as a human being. Thus the organisation delineates what are considered to be officially appropriate standards of welfare, joint values, incentives and penalties.

(Goffman, 1961: p.164)

These standards, values, carrots and sticks need to be articulated. For nurses the first step is through the selection or development of a model appropriate to practice, management and research.

References

Collister B   1986   Psychiatric nursing and a developmental model. In *Models for Nursing*, B Kershaw & J Salvage (Eds). John Wiley & Sons, Chichester.

Fitzpatrick J & Whall A   1983   *Conceptual Models of Nursing. Analysis and Application*. Robert J Brady Co, Bowie, Maryland.

Goffman I   1961   *Asylums* (1968 Edition). Penguin, London.

Riehl JP & Roy C   1980   *Conceptual Models in Nursing Practice*. Appleton-Century-Crofts, New York.

Index